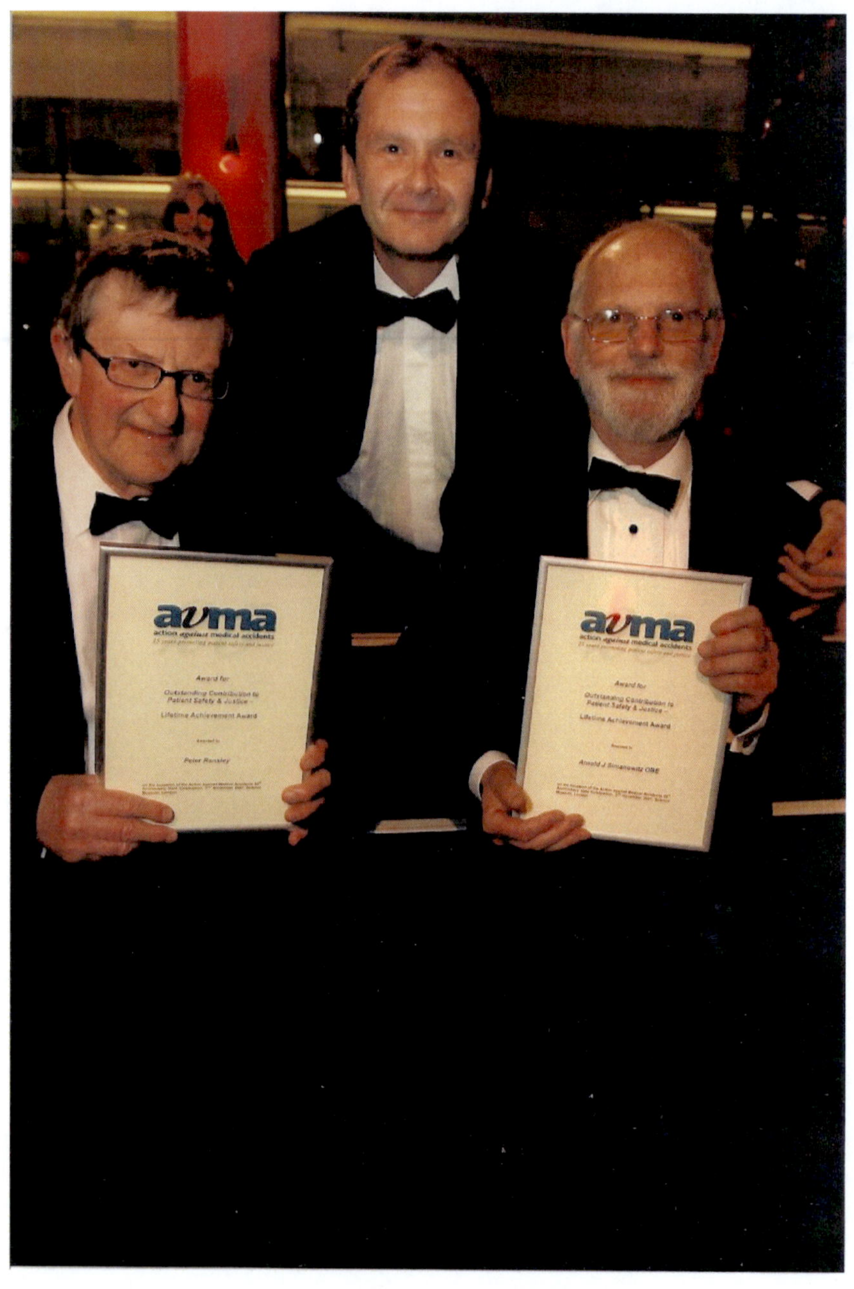


L-R first Chief Executive Arnold Simanowitz and his successor Peter Walsh
at AvMA's 25th anniversary celebration 2007.

# The Man Under the Clapham Omnibus

## (The search for patient safety and justice)

### Arnold Simanowitz

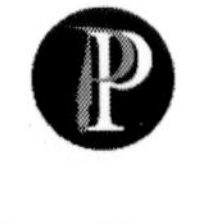

Pen Press

First published in Great Britain by Pen Press

All paper used in the printing of this book has been made from wood grown in managed, sustainable forests.

ISBN13: 978-1-78003-544-4

Printed and bound in the UK
Pen Press is an imprint of
Indepenpress Publishing Limited
25 Eastern Place
Brighton
BN2 1GJ

A catalogue record of this book is available from
the British Library

Cover design by Jacqueline Abromeit

# Contents

# Acknowledgements

There are a number of people to whom I would like to acknowledge my indebtedness. Firstly Peter Ransley, the inspiration and founder of AVMA. It was he who gave me the chance to make the contribution I have made and more importantly, although AVMA was in effect his baby, allowed me the freedom to build the organisation whilst always being a fount of ideas and support. He retired as Chair in 1988 and because of his contribution was unanimously elected as Honorary Life President. He was succeeded by Derek Kartun. Derek was wise and politically astute and throughout his term gave me both excellent support and helpful advice, ensuring, when necessary, that the Board of Trustees maintained a realistic understanding of what we could achieve. Derek was followed by Barbara Banks in 1995. Barbara, a Professor of Physiological Chemistry, had herself been a victim of a medical accident. Although she fought and lost (unfairly in her and our view) a costly legal action to try and recover compensation for the permanent damage she had suffered she was nevertheless able to maintain a balanced view of the medical profession many of whom had been taught by her over the years. As a result she was able to bring a unique insight into the problems and needs of victims and she too was a major support to me and influence on AVMA's success.

I started writing this book shortly after my retirement from AVMA in 2002. Unfortunately I found that I soon became as busy in "retirement" as I had been while working for AVMA and whilst I continued to write whenever I had a moment it was not until 2012 that I began to concentrate fully on completing the book. By that time, nearly ten years after my retirement, my memory for details had obviously become less acute. Nevertheless I have tried to make the history of the organisation as comprehensive as possible. What may have happened, however, is that I may have omitted to mention some people who made a significant contribution to the development of both AVMA and medical negligence litigation. If I have inadvertently done so I would like them to accept my sincere apologies. The creation and success of AVMA was always a team effort and I hope that this comes through in the pages of this book.

# Foreword by
# James Badenoch QC

This book has a remarkable author, and it tells a remarkable story of a tiny, fledgling and underfunded charity which grew into an organisation of national importance, and became a major force for good.

Arnold Simanowitz was imbued by his early life under apartheid in his native South Africa with hatred for injustice and with a compassion for its victims which impelled him to use his energy and his formidable intellect in their cause. Having become a lawyer, and settled in the UK, he would certainly have found success and financial security in conventional legal practice. Fortunately for us he found instead the cause he was to fight for, and to which thereafter he devoted his life until his retirement, marked by the well-deserved award of the OBE, in 2002. The cause was "Action for Victims of Medical Accidents", AVMA, as it was named at its birth, and this book is his account of the passion which drove him and of the twenty-year journey on which that passion took him.

It becomes painfully clear that AVMA's name reflected a shameful truth of those times. Patients injured by medical accidents, even those crippled physically and financially, were all too often very ill-served or not served at all by the professionals upon whose help they should have been able to rely. The medical profession frequently abandoned them, and the lawyers enlisted by them were frequently supine in the face of the myriad obstacles and traps in the way of anyone foolish or daring enough to embark on medical litigation.

So it was that AVMA was formed by Arnold, the playwright Peter Ransley, and a small group of determined supporters, to confront the victimhood of these unfortunates, and as the early chapters show "victim" was certainly the right description. They were victims of the cost of litigation and its innumerable delays; of barriers to obtaining notes and records and even basic medical information about their case; of doctors' unwillingness to break ranks and give impartial evidence against a colleague; of unfair and prejudicial rules of civil litigation with no pre-trial exchange of expert reports; of an automatic, implacable and often aggressive resistance by medical defendants' advisers to all claims however meritorious; and perhaps most regrettably of antipathy and even outright hostility from judges to claims against medical professionals. Added to this shaming list was a general ignorance and lack of experience on the part of most lawyers in respect of medical cases and how to go about them, with their resultant tendency to freeze like a rabbit in the headlights when clinical litigation was contemplated. To the dismal truth of this picture I can personally attest, with bitter memories of my early experience as a young barrister practising in the field (my case of Dobbie, referred to in the book, is engraved on my heart). AVMA had many battles to fight.

Happily, and he writes of himself, Arnold was "able to see the problems of medical accidents in perspective from the victims' point of view". With that perspective (which so many at the time conspicuously lacked), and an iron will cloaked in old-world courtesy, Arnold galvanised his devoted team at AVMA to tackle the system's injustices and inadequacies, and to reform outmoded attitudes among lawyers and doctors. He describes how a panel was established of solicitors provenly expert in clinical litigation, which has served to exclude from practice in the field all but those with relevant specialist experience; how a Lawyers' Support Group was set up to educate and advise lawyers in relevant matters; and how a Lawyers' Service was inaugurated to collate and provide the names of trustworthy and impartial expert witnesses for medico-legal opinion. Above all the founding principle of AVMA has been constantly upheld by a dedicated Casework Department which delivers help, support and guidance without charge to injured patients who need and seek its help.

The notable success of these efforts makes for a happy ending to this book. It has enabled the charity to widen its focus and to take on the leading role which it has for some time so effectively played in improving risk management and patient safety – the prevention of victimhood. That it has seemed right now to change the name to AvMA (Action **against** Medical Accidents) under

Peter Walsh, Arnold's worthy successor as Chief Executive who contributes the closing chapter to the book, truly reflects that success – as does the fact that the medical profession, once largely hostile to all AVMA stood for, has come to recognise the good it has done and to welcome and support its work.

This is the story of AVMA, wonderfully and entertainingly told. I commend it to everyone, professional and lay, who has anything to do with medicine, which means all of us at some time in our lives. We owe a debt of gratitude to Arnold Simanowitz and to all who have worked for and supported AVMA, for what it stood for, and for what it achieved, and for what, as AvMA, it continues to achieve. This book will tell you why that is so.

# Foreword by
# Harvey Marcovitch FRCP Hon FRCPCH, Paediatrician

Twenty-five years ago I dipped into what was probably a highly irregular bank account, held in the name of my hospital department, to enable a mother of a multiply disabled child to attend a conference on cerebral palsy. The objective for disposing of our slush fund in this way was to assist her in understanding the incurable nature of her child's condition, something which her doctors, by confusing her with euphemisms, had failed to do. The result was not as intended. At the conference (or in the bar?) she met a feisty solicitor, one Arnold Simanowitz, who told her that a major problem faced by the infant AvMA was the unhelpfulness of doctors. "I'm sure my doctor would help," she told him. The innocent sounding letter that followed from Arnold only flattered to deceive. In consenting to offer him advice from time to time it did not occur to me that this would provoke an avalanche of requests from solicitors, hitherto thwarted in their attempts to seek an objective expert opinion.

Nowadays, many of my younger colleagues express irritation or anger at what they perceive as the multiple jeopardy in which they stand, their acts and omissions potentially scrutinised by their employers, their regulatory body, the civil and criminal justice systems and the Press. Despite much scientific evidence to the contrary, they find it hard to accept that so few of their errors will provoke investigation or litigation and that when they do the burden of proof serves to protect them.

When I first encountered AVMA, solicitors were often groping in the dark, case notes were often not fully disclosed, allegations were imprecise, schedules non-existent, and many experts were part of a regiment of hired guns who appeared to care more for their fees than the accuracy of their advice. Even those doing their best to be objective flew largely by the seat of their pants without the clarity of Civil Procedure Rules to guide them.

It is an enormous tribute to the progenitors of AVMA that so much has changed, an arduous process detailed with enthusiasm and humour in this book. It is an embarrassing lesson that so little of the progress was headed or supported by my fellow medical professionals but a comfort that sheer persistence by the author and his associates has led to changes in the behaviour of medical defence bodies and the General Medical Council, however grudgingly conceded, a far higher standard of performance by lawyers and a more generous spirit from those administering funds available for legal aid, albeit that the last is now under threat.

Life may be easier for potential litigants than it was in 1980 but so much more is still needed. My experience as an expert witness, an adjudicator for the Medical Practitioners Tribunal Service (previously GMC Fitness to Practise) and an adviser to a number of inquiries into medical misfortunes tells me that the healthcare system struggles with being open and honest when its employees have transgressed and is yet to find adequate ways to learn from its mistakes. The medical profession would do well to understand the history of AVMA as portrayed by Arnold Simanowitz and take heed of the campaigns that surely remain, as described in this book by Peter Walsh, AvMA CEO.

# Chapter 1
# First stirrings

I first expressed interest in the politics of change at the age of ten through humour. It was 1948 and campaigning in the General Election in South Africa where I was born was taking place. It was a vicious campaign, particularly on the part of the opposition Nationalist Party (known colloquially as the Nats) who were determined if elected to introduce their policy of apartheid. (Their slogan for the election was "Stem wit, stem Nat." – Vote white, vote Nat.)

This did not of course stop the media, as they are wont to do wherever a reasonably free media exists, also reporting on trivia. My mother read out a newspaper headline reporting that General Smuts (the Prime Minister at the time) had been stung by a wasp. Sweetly and innocently I enquired whether "they were sure it wasn't a g(nat)".

It was not surprising that even at that age I was aware of the strong feelings my parents had against the Nationalists. They were living in Oudtshoorn when I was born. This was a small town in the Afrikaner hinterland of the Cape Province where my paternal grandparents had settled when they emigrated from Poland in 1905. It had achieved fame for fifteen minutes in the early part of the century as the centre of the ostrich feather boom. Many Jewish refugees from the pogroms of Eastern Europe were attracted to Oudtshoorn at that time and notwithstanding their unlikely backgrounds established themselves as ostrich farmers.

Not my grandfather. He was a Yeshivabocher – a perpetual student of Judaism and the bible – and made a few pounds as a Hebrew teacher and assistant at the synagogue. It was my grandmother who supported the family. Notwithstanding her nine children she managed to run a small general dealers from which she eked out just about a sufficient living for the family to survive.

My father was the eldest male and notwithstanding that his ambition was to be a doctor and he had already started medical school, his parents persuaded him that it was his duty to run the family business. It turned out that he had a flair for this and within a few years the business had grown substantially and, under the name Wholesale Retailers, had become the largest general dealer in the town with a strong reputation.

But it was now 1943 and South Africa was heavily involved in the war on the side of the Allies. This was not popular with a large section of the Afrikaners. Many identified with the racial purity ideas of the Nazis while others simply wanted the Germans to win so as to get rid of the hated English. The more extreme among them banded themselves into secret and not-so-secret societies such as the Ossewa Brandwag (oxwaggon firewatch), which carried out attacks on Jews and Jewish properties. This organisation in fact had a shop front on the high street in Oudtshoorn which proudly sported the swastika. One night my father was woken in the middle of the night because his shop was on fire. He dashed to the scene where a whole row of Jewish shops were alight. Not a particularly emotional man, he stood in the road and wept as he watched a life's work slowly go up in flames while an antiquated and inadequate fire service which had taken its time to arrive could do nothing to halt the conflagration.

For the rest of his life my father never spoke to me or my siblings of the disaster. I moved to England when I was twenty-two and saw him only on the rare trips I made to visit him in Cape Town. On my penultimate visit, when he was ninety-three and apparently in full possession of his faculties save for being almost stone deaf, I felt it was important to capture his recollections of his life before it was too late. I began to interview him on video. He responded well until I began asking him about the fire. "How much do you remember about the fire in Oudtshoorn?" I enquired. "What fire?" "The one that burnt down your shop." "My shop wasn't burnt down." "Don't you remember Wholesale Retailers was burnt down and they said it was the Ossewa Brandwag that did it?" "No."

Following the fire my parents decided that it would be better to move to Cape Town where my mother had been born and brought up and where they had family and friends. Whilst my father had been influenced by the culture and attitudes of small town Afrikanerdom my mother had been exposed to the progressive ideas of a city which, being an important port, had always practised a modicum of internationalism. Indeed in her youth she had flirted with Communism and whilst she soon dropped that for the ambitions of marriage and home-making, prevalent among the majority of South African white women, she retained a strong sense of justice and egalitarianism which proved to be the major influence in my life.

I turned five two months after we arrived in Cape Town. My father had been severely affected by the fire and gradually showed less and less interest in family affairs and least of all in me. It was this, and the fact that I was my mother's favourite (or believed myself to be – in later years it transpired that my older brother believed the same about himself) that meant that it was my mother's values that I adopted.

My life, as I grew up, was full of contradictions. We were certainly not a rich family by the usual white standards. After the fire in Oudtshoorn we moved to Cape Town and my father tried a number of businesses without much success. It seemed that the drive had gone out of him. Eventually he settled into a shop, which he called Cranfords, which combined the sale of antiques with second-hand books. Whilst, at least with regard to the books side, the shop developed a national if not an international reputation it was not highly profitable.

Nevertheless I lived a privileged life. We had an adequate house in Camps Bay, a seaside suburb of Cape Town. I have since travelled to many of the beauty spots of the world, but Camps Bay, nestling under Table Mountain and right on the sea, I consider to be one of the most beautiful places in the world. My house was a hundred yards from the beach with a sweeping view of the bay. In summer the reflection of the sun on the slowly shifting deep blue sea, which ebbed and flowed onto the sand which had a whiteness that detergent manufacturers would have died for, had a magic attraction for me from an early age. My most nostalgic memories of my late teens, however, are of sitting on the verandah on a summer's evening as the sun went down and watching the sky change into such a fantastic kaleidoscope of colour that it was almost painful to keep my eyes on it.

Against this idyll was the ever-present knowledge of the conditions in which the non-white people lived. How much did that impinge on my life? As a young child, I must confess, not a lot. Partly this must have been because of the sheer joy of the life I was living. How many young children revelling in the near perfect life of the white South African in idyllic surroundings would stop to think how unfair it was that not everybody could enjoy that life? The contradictions were even more evident in the behaviour of my mother. She was a voracious reader and had read amongst others all the Left Book Club books which, right until I left South Africa, graced the top shelf of our bookcase in the hall. In any political discussion she vigorously maintained an anti-apartheid position and expressed sympathy with the suffering of black people. Yet our succession of black maids – we were not too poor to be unable to afford a maid at the miserable wage that all black workers received – were obliged to live in an outside room which not only was perpetually damp but had no electricity or running water. The maid was not allowed to use our bath but had to use a tin tub which she filled in the kitchen and then had to heave into her room.

As I grew up I became more aware of these contradictions and more political. I became imbued with the idea of equality for all people and pained by the suffering of the black majority. The Nationalists had swept into power in 1948 and gradually introduced more and more restrictions on the black population, causing greater and greater hardship and suffering. The opposition United Party, which at best wished to temper this hardship without granting the black population any rights, offered nothing to those like me who wanted to see real change. There were of course those who clandestinely belonged to or supported the proscribed Communist party or the Liberal Party which, though a capitalist party, believed in immediate equal rights for all and were prepared to face prison themselves in demonstrating for their principles.

By the age of 18 I was fully committed to all the ideas of the Liberal party and much of what the Communist Party stood for. I suppose if someone had given me a label at that time I would have been called a socialist. I did not, however, join either the Communists or the Liberals. There were two reasons for this. Firstly I had not been sufficiently exposed to their ideas. Unlike many of my contemporaries I had not gone to university full time. It was there, as in all universities, that students had the time both to read and discuss the great issues of the day and indeed to be influenced by any enlightened tutors who might be around. For mainly financial reasons I had gone straight from school into a law office to become articled to an attorney, a five-year training commitment. Not that I was paid a fortune for working there – in the first three months I received nothing and in the following year £3 per month. Of course my parents were saved the university fees which were substantially greater than the part-time evening studies that I had to undertake. To give my parents their due they did make it clear that if I had definite ideas about what I wanted to study they would have tried to make the sacrifices necessary to send me to university.

But I was not at all clear about what I wanted to study or indeed what I wanted to be. I went into the law by default and under the influence of my uncle who was a successful attorney. Not only did he influence my taking up the law but he convinced my parents that if I was going to be an attorney it would be a waste of time my studying for a law degree. Far better to obtain the practical experience gained from five years of articles. As a person with a strong pragmatic approach to life that practical approach did appeal to me.

In the absence of the influence of university life, and given my pragmatism, when a group of opposition members of parliament broke away from the United Party in 1959 to form the Progressive Party I was immediately attracted to it. The main thrust of that party's policies was the gradual granting of equal rights to the black population through a qualified franchise. It would immediately get rid of the petty apartheid legislation but the acquiring of the vote would depend on a combination of property ownership and education. Looking back today, I do cringe at the idea that it would still be the white population granting the black population rights to which they were entitled as of right. My excuse today is that this was the first time that a white party, with parliamentary representatives, was prepared to acknowledge the basic equality of black people in South Africa. It was of course a compromise, but not of my principles. I truly believed that, at that time, other than through revolution the only way in which the black population would achieve equal rights was by persuading the white population to grant them.

And so I joined the Progressives, becoming, at the age of 18, one of their first secretaries of a parliamentary constituency. I still possess the Party card that was issued to me in 1959. I like to think that with Helen Suzman, who for years following the first elections after the break with the United Party, was the only MP from the Progressives, I was at least in good company.

In 1960 the opposition by the black population against the hated pass laws reached a critical stage. There were mass demonstrations all over the country. During March there was wide campaigning in the townships, and on the 21st March the Sharpeville massacre took place when the police shot and killed 69 demonstrators. Partly in response to that there was rioting in the Cape Town townships and on the 30th March the government declared a State of Emergency. Both the Pan Africanist Congress and the African National Congress (ANC), the two major rival political movements representing the black population, were banned and hundreds were brutally arrested.

Later on that day I was in my office when the husband of one of our secretaries burst in and announced that thousands of blacks had assembled outside the Magistrates' Court. That was less than half a mile from my office and of course a place with which I was very familiar and I decided to go and have a look. When I arrived there were indeed thousands (later reported to have been 30,000) gathered in an entirely peaceful demonstration. There appeared to be some negotiation with the police taking place and as there was no other action I returned to my office after about an hour.

The next day I learned that the police had agreed with the leader of the demonstration, Peter Kgosana, that if he told the crowd to return peacefully to their townships he would be able to meet the Minister of Justice. He had agreed to this and the crowd had peacefully dispersed. The police then arrested Kgosana and the government ordered the army to place a ring of steel around the townships so that no further demonstrations could take place, and at the same time hundreds of further arrests of "troublemakers" took place. These incidents had a profound effect on me. I recall a discussion with a number of friends when we speculated what we would do if we were called up into the army to take part in the containing of the townships. I knew that I would have to refuse, whatever the consequences.

The repression of the black population intensified after that but the government was, through that repression, able to maintain some kind of peace in the country. The reaction of the world to the Sharpeville massacre, however, prompted the South African Government to pursue its ideal of becoming a Republic so that any vestige of control by Britain could be terminated. The next months were quite tumultuous in the history of South Africa. For me the first priority was to ensure that it did not become a Republic so that whatever restraining influence of Britain was retained. To this end I was heavily involved in campaigning for a "No" vote in the Referendum held on the 5th October 1960. During the campaigning the Prime Minister, Dr Verwoerd, assured the country that becoming a republic would not mean that South Africa would leave the Commonwealth. That had some influence on the result of the referendum which went in the government's favour by the small majority of 52% to 47%. As a result of the referendum, plans were made by the government to declare a Republic on the 31st May 1961. In March 1961, Verwoerd visited the Imperial Conference in London to discuss South Africa becoming a republic within the Commonwealth. As the status of South Africa would change, he had to submit an application for a renewal of its membership of the Commonwealth.

In the light of the attacks on apartheid by both a number of Commonwealth leaders and campaigners in Britain and around the world it became almost certain that South Africa's application would be rejected. In order to save face Dr Verwoerd, on 15 March 1961, withdrew the application, arguing that the Commonwealth had no right to question and criticise the domestic affairs of his country. He announced that South Africa would become a republic outside the Commonwealth. So despite the assurances given by the government during the referendum, assurances which probably led to the victory of the "yes" campaign, it withdrew South Africa from the Commonwealth.

In the meantime, on the 14th February 1961 I qualified as an attorney and my firm offered me a partnership. This was extremely tempting as I had had a steady girlfriend for some years and wanted to marry her. So, notwithstanding my concerns about the way the country was going, I accepted. It was agreed however that I would first have a six-week holiday in Europe. My boss, and potential partner had only reluctantly agreed to this. He could not understand why I felt I needed to go. When, in an attempt to explain, I pointed out that it was axiomatic that travel broadens the mind his reply was that he had never travelled and to look at who he was! Eventually he did agree and in June 1961, just nine days after the proclamation of the Republic of South Africa, I sailed to England.

England was a revelation to me. The people I met, the newspapers I read and the general atmosphere hit me almost like an electric shock and highlighted for me both the provincialism and the repressive nature of the society for all people, black and white, in South Africa. I had not left as a political escapee but after just two weeks in England I felt that I could not make my life, and certainly could not bring up children, in South Africa. I was due to hitchhike round Europe with a friend during my holiday and by the time I got to Belgium, having additionally been exposed to a great diversity of young people in the youth hostels in which I had stayed, it became clear to me that I would not return to South Africa to live. I remember sitting on a kerbstone in Brussels and writing letters both to my parents and my firm informing them. I am not sure who got the bigger shock but I know my mother was extremely distressed. Nevertheless she did not criticise me, as basically she agreed with my reasons.

This book is not meant to be a detailed memoir of my life but I do wish to show the influences which led to the cementing of my ambition to help the underdog and which culminated in my setting up the charity Action for Victims of Medical Accidents (AVMA). I therefore deal very shortly with my life from then until I became involved in AVMA.

The few weeks I spent travelling in Europe continued to open my eyes as I met more young people from many different countries. So many of them seemed to have such an exciting and open view of the world compared to my friends back home. Only one incident showed me that perhaps I was looking only for the positives and becoming a bit starry-eyed. Lying in the dark one night in a dormitory in a Youth Hostel in Germany I heard someone fart loudly. In response I heard clearly, although uttered sotto voce, "*Verdammte Jude!*"

From Europe I travelled by boat to Israel. By then I was becoming more interested in socialism as a result not only of my contact with fellow travellers (in the true sense of the words!) but also my increasingly long discussions with Val, my future wife, whom I had met in Athens. I was in no way a Zionist but I did have some interest in seeing the Jewish "homeland". My main reason for going to Israel was, however, to experience what I understood to be a pure form of socialism on a kibbutz. I may not have experienced pure socialism – the ideals of the founders of the kibbutz were becoming much watered down by both the influences of capitalism and the disillusionment of the younger generation – but I did experience pure love in my relationship with Val. So after six months in Israel we returned to England to marry and to live.

Once back in England I decided that if I wanted to pursue a career in the Law, and not waste the legal qualification I had worked so hard to achieve in South Africa, I had to re-qualify as a solicitor in the English jurisdiction. The two jurisdictions were of course very different, South African law being mainly based on Roman-Dutch law and English law being based on the Common Law of England. The truth is that, because of the major differences in the two systems, South African lawyers should have been required to undergo the full training required by English residents starting from scratch. However, because most Commonwealth countries based their law on English law, there was a significant exemption for all Commonwealth lawyers who were only required to work as a bona fide clerk in a solicitors' office for two years and pass Part 2 of the Solicitors' Qualifying Examination to become admitted as a solicitor in England. That was instead of having to undertake five years' articles of clerkship as well as passing Part 1 and 2 of the exam.

But South Africa was no longer a Commonwealth member. Fortunately for me, the regulations surrounding South Africa's departure from the Commonwealth had provided, at least in the case of recognition of legal qualifications, that the exemptions would continue to apply for one year from that departure. That meant as long as I was in employment in a solicitor's office as a "bona fide clerk" on the 31st May 1962 the exemption would apply to me. As Val and I had landed in England on the 26th May there followed a desperate search for a firm that would take me on. After numerous applications I finally secured an interview with Sidney Hackman & Co. in the West End. The interview did not go promisingly. Mr Hackman explained that he needed someone to run his litigation department and without the experience of English practice I would not be able to cope. I got up to leave with a sinking feeling – it was only one day to go to the deadline after which, if I wanted to re-qualify, I would have to do three years' articles as well as all the exams. Desperation made me bold. I turned to Mr Hackman: "Your advertisement has been with the Law Society for more than nine months," I said, "how are you going to manage?" He replied that it was extremely difficult. I then suggested to him that taking me on would not be worse than having nobody. I would surely be able to do something. I explained why I had to be in employment on the 31st May and even if he paid me a nominal salary and it did not work out we would have helped each other. Much to my delight he agreed and offered me what I thought was a generous salary in the circumstances – £12 per week. I spent the next four years running the litigation department of Sidney Hackman & Company in the West End and the final two of those years studying part-time for the Part 2 exam. This was a means to an end. I was determined to use my skills and knowledge other than acting for car hire firms, landlords and the like.

Towards the end of my time with Sidney Hackman, and having sat for, but not yet having received the results of the Part 2 examination, Val and I decided that we wanted to experience an independent African country for ourselves. This was particularly important for me having come from the oppression of South Africa where newspapers daily carried reports of the disasters that followed independence in African countries. Val had been a supporter of anti-apartheid for years. I applied for and secured a position as a solicitor in Livingstone in Zambia to run a branch office of what was then the largest firm of solicitors in Africa, Ellis & Co. As soon as I learned that I had passed the exam and had become admitted as a solicitor, we set sail for Cape Town from where we travelled by train to Livingstone. It was on that journey that an incident occurred that was to determine how I was going to conduct my life in future.

The train from Cape Town stopped in Bulawayo in what was then Southern Rhodesia governed by Ian Smith's illegal government. As the train was to remain there for some hours Val and I decided to take a taxi into town to look around. In the taxi I got chatting to the African driver and told him where I was going and what I was going to do. On returning to the station after a few hours I noticed a large crowd of Africans gathered around the entrance to the platform through which Val and I had to pass. I must confess to a frisson of fear, caused no doubt by my background in South Africa. As we passed, however I heard muttering among the crowd. As it was repeated I was eventually able to make out what they were saying. "It's the defender, he's the defender," they were saying to each other. It was for me like a sudden illumination. Yes, I was going to be a defender. That was my destiny.

In Livingstone, being in control of a branch office, and the only solicitor there, I had to do all kinds of work but I certainly enjoyed most the defending of Africans charged with all kinds of offences. It was at times quite scary as there was no division between barristers and solicitors so I often found myself appearing in the High Court for men charged with murder. As Zambia still had the death penalty I felt a huge responsibility. Fortunately I never had to see the judge put on his black cap. We were in Zambia for nearly three years and found it very satisfying. I was developing the practice and Val had secured a job as teacher in a secondary school. We had also become involved with South African ANC exiles who were training to start a military resistance against the regime. I knew, however, that I wanted more out of legal practice.

During our time in Zambia we drove on holiday down to Cape Town where my parents still lived. One day I was lying on the beach chatting to my close friend Henry Brown. He had remained working in South Africa and had become the attorney for many of the ANC members who were being harassed by the police. In fact he had represented Nelson Mandela in a number of matters while he was incarcerated on Robben Island. Henry felt, however, that because of the increasing repression by the government it was becoming harder and harder to help and he wanted to leave South Africa. We hatched plans to set up in law together one day, somewhere in the world where we could develop a radical practice that would make a contribution to freedom and justice.

Unfortunately Val's and my time in Zambia was tragically brought to a premature end. Our second child, born in Zambia and only 11 months old, fell ill with extreme diarrhoea and was admitted to the local hospital. At the time we were harbouring two South African guerrillas and feeling hugely pleased that we were doing our small bit to change things down south. At two o'clock in the morning we received a call to come to the hospital urgently. On arrival we saw our little Aidan struggling for breath and the doctor informed us that he had little hope of surviving. We had only been there about half an hour when he died. We returned home in a state of absolute shock and despair. The South Africans were incredibly sympathetic and understanding and immediately agreed that they could no longer stay with us. They departed and we collapsed into grief.

We both found it too distressing to remain in Zambia. Coming there had been a great and exciting adventure but now everywhere we went, everything we did was tinged with deep sadness. Within a month, in June 1969, we had both left our jobs and returned to England.

While I had been in Zambia, a friend of mine, Gerald Heiman, had written to me about the possibility of my joining him in a practice in South London which he had recently purchased. At that time I was not thinking of leaving Zambia but I replied that I might be interested when I did return. When we hastily left Zambia I contacted him and joined him in the firm, Armstrong & Co, initially as an assistant and then as a partner. Whilst I was able to do a lot of legal aid work there I still nurtured the ambition of using my legal training to do more for society. When Henry Brown eventually left South Africa and settled in England we were able to revive our ideas about setting up together.

In 1975 I left Armstrongs (having first ensured that yet another South African friend, who had emigrated to England, was a replacement acceptable to Gerald). Henry and I established a firm, Simanowitz & Brown, in Waterloo. Our somewhat ambitious aim was to act and seek justice for the disadvantaged and provide the kind of top class service for them that was usually reserved for the rich. Without compromising our principles we would use the more lucrative side of the law to subsidise the work that hardly paid. Henry was an accomplished commercial lawyer and also had a clientele of South African refugee organisations. For my sins my responsibilities included the domestic conveyancing, although that was only because Henry knew even less about conveyancing than I did. We did have fun practising together as we got on so well. It was just as well because I recall a big laugh over something that could have been a major disaster. I was acting for a South African liberation organisation on their purchase of a property. The day before completion was due they brought in a Bank Draft for the balance of the purchase price, £25,000.

Later in the day when I was preparing for completion I could not find the draft. Panic set in. Both Henry and I searched the office but drew a blank. I remembered that it had been brought in while I was opening the post. Henry dashed downstairs just before the dustman arrived, trawled through the dustbin – and found it. Only very good friends could have had a laugh about that.

Notwithstanding the fun we were having, and, I believe, the good we were doing, we found it more and more difficult, however hard we worked, to make the practice pay. One of the major problems was that the Legal Aid Board was becoming increasingly mean with its payments. As at least half of our work was legal aid work I found myself having to work twice as hard for half the money. (The shrinking band of solicitors still doing legal aid work now would probably consider that in my day legal aid was a sinecure.) In responding to a survey into legal aid at the time, we quoted Lewis Carroll's red queen:

"It takes all the running you can do to stay in the same place. If you want to get somewhere else, you have to run twice as fast."

Eventually the monthly scramble to maintain solvency began to tell on both Henry and me and we decided that we either had to become more commercial or sell the practice and go our own way. I was already feeling that since my epiphany on the way to Zambia I had made too many compromises and I was not prepared to adopt the first option. As with all the decisions we had made throughout our partnership we amicably agreed to sell.

What to do next? To explain that I have to go back in time a little.

# Chapter 2
# The founding of
# Action for the Victims of Medical Accidents
# AVMA

In 1979 an article appeared in the *New Statesman* about a woman who had been through a torrid time in hospital as a result of a botched sterilisation. It related not only the trauma of the accident but also the difficulty she had had finding out what had happened and seeking compensation for the quite severe disability with which she had been left. This was the story of Stella Burnett which at that time used a different name to preserve her anonymity.

This article was drawn to the attention of Peter Ransley, an up-and-coming playwright, who found the story so intriguing and disturbing that he wrote a play for television, Minor Complications, which dramatically told Stella's story. The play showed how she underwent a "simple" procedure, a laparoscopic sterilisation, during which her bowel was punctured. After the operation she became steadily more ill but nurses and doctors refused to contemplate that anything serious was wrong and preferred to believe that Stella was a somewhat hysterical woman unused to a little pain.

The play was a superb reconstruction of events, showing the anxiety and then desperation of Stella, her friends and family, as she gradually deteriorated, while the medical establishment closed their minds to the possibility that anything had gone wrong. Others were not so complacent. A friend of Stella's, a radiotherapist, was so concerned that she kept notes of what she saw when she visited. These notes proved extremely useful to Peter when he was writing the play. Eventually, Stella became so ill that even the doctors had to acknowledge that all was not right. A surgeon from another team was called and he immediately realised that Stella was in extreme danger. She was rushed to the operating theatre and re-opened. The surgeon discovered that her bowel had been punctured during the laparoscopy and had become gangrenous. The only way he could save Stella was to remove a large part of it.

Over time, Stella recovered, but with a substantial piece of her large intestine removed she was never going to be fully well. She continued to suffer from pain and intestinal problems, lost her job and found it hard to look after her two small children. She also suffered considerable psychological effects. As her physical and mental strength returned she began to think of finding out what had happened and why. Friends encouraged her also to think about seeking compensation as, unable to work, she was in a pretty poor financial position.

Her first letter of enquiry addressed to the hospital was met, after many weeks, with an apology that she was left in a bad way but no explanation whatsoever. Further letters elicited nothing better. So she turned to the law. She approached a solicitor who had conducted her conveyancing work some time previously. He had no experience in dealing with a case of alleged medical negligence. Without checking on the medical background, or seeking a medical expert's opinion, he fired off a letter demanding an explanation and compensation.

Again after a considerable lapse of time (during which the solicitor took no further action) a reply was received denying liability. The solicitor realised it was not going to be as simple as he had thought. So finance was the next problem. Any litigation costs a lot. Medical negligence litigation could cost many thousands of pounds. The solicitor applied for legal aid on behalf of his client. It was refused on the basis that the solicitor had not shown that there was a case that would justify the granting of legal aid. That was not surprising as the solicitor had not obtained the medical records nor the advice of a medical expert to show that there was potentially a good case.

Unusually the solicitor decided to continue with the case on a paying basis without demanding a large sum of money in advance. He had problems obtaining the medical records: the hospital solicitors were obstructive and it took many months before they disclosed them. Finally, however, the solicitor found himself in a position to instruct a doctor to obtain an expert opinion on the cause of Stella's problems. He chose a doctor whom the firm had used for other accident work. Notwithstanding that it appeared to the solicitor to be an open-and-shut case, the medical expert reported that there was no negligence. According to him the kind of accident that had happened was unavoidable so there was no fault on the part of the surgeon, that is, no negligence, and therefore no claim. The report did not attempt to explain how the accident had occurred.

Stella did not give up. She could not believe that she could have gone in for a straightforward minor operation, could have suffered so much damage and yet there was no explanation for what had happened, why it had happened and who, if anyone, was to blame. She began to think the unthinkable – that the medical profession was covering up. She was told about a doctor who might be sympathetic. When she met him he did indeed seem sympathetic, and the report he produced did seem to suggest that something had gone wrong. But it nevertheless concluded that there had been no negligence.

Again, while the solicitor said that on the basis of that report they would have to accept that it was not going to be possible to prove negligence, Stella was not satisfied. She decided to try to understand the medical issues herself. She went to the library and researched the operation in detail until she felt she had a good understanding of the medical procedure. Looking at the report in the light of her new knowledge it seemed to her that the expert had clearly indicated that the surgeon had been at fault, yet he was still saying that there had been no negligence.

She and her solicitor returned to the expert. She put her conclusions to him. He agreed with her. She asked him whether that did not mean that the surgeon had been negligent. He again agreed that it did. Stella was amazed. The expert was prepared to make an honest appraisal of what had gone wrong but he had not been prepared to follow the logic of his assessment and say in writing that the gynaecologist had been negligent. Having been confronted by Stella with a straight question, however, he gave a straight answer. That was a major breakthrough. Now all it needed was for her solicitor to put that evidence to the defendants and negotiate a settlement.

But that was not quite what happened next. Her solicitor, who had been working for years on the case without asking for money, now wanted a substantial deposit before he went any further.

Stella had been lucky that she had got so far without finance. Having been refused legal aid, normally a victim of medical negligence without substantial means of her own would simply have had to give up. Stella had hoped that her solicitor would have waited to be paid once she had been successful. She had not allowed herself to think what would happen if she were unsuccessful.

Clearly her solicitor was suddenly doing just that. Notwithstanding that the case was now more hopeful than it had ever been, he had obviously realised the risk he had been taking and was not prepared to continue with the case unless he had some cover for his costs. As will have been gathered, Stella was not one to give up, especially now that she felt herself so close to victory. She approached a number of contacts that she thought might be prepared to help. One of them, having heard the whole story, realised that it was now not so great a gamble and agreed to lend her the deposit.

Armed with the expert's report, Stella's solicitor approached the doctor's solicitors. Although until then they had denied emphatically that their client had done anything wrong, they were suddenly prepared to negotiate. Soon they agreed to pay Stella the princely sum of £25,000. £25,000 to compensate for the almost unbearable pain and suffering she had undergone; for the crippling condition with which she had been left for life; to compensate for the earnings she had lost over three years and the damage to her career. Yet she could not afford to litigate further and at least she was getting some financial compensation plus the satisfaction that the doctor had been shown to have been negligent. Whether he, or the hospital, would have learned anything as a result of the claim is another matter.

When Peter wrote the play he thought he was dealing with an isolated, albeit shocking, incident. He was not prepared for what happened after the play was shown as Play for Today on BBC 1 in 1980. The BBC received hundreds of letters from people who had watched the play. Furthermore, as Action Lines did not exist at the BBC at that time Peter had left his home telephone number at the duty desk. As a result, in addition to the letters he received a large number of phone calls. These contacts identified wholly with the victim in the play. Many of them told heartrending stories of the loss of loved ones, children who had been brain damaged and had suffered other serious consequences. All of them believed that they or their relative had had a medical accident; all of them had tried to get an explanation but had met with a wall of silence; and none of them had received adequate or any compensation.

Peter realised that he had stumbled on a social problem of potentially enormous proportions. He felt unable to ignore it. So he wrote to the *Guardian* saying that he thought that an organisation was needed to help people who had suffered in that way. He asked anyone who was interested in assisting to contact him. Now I had not seen the play and had not read the letter page of the *Guardian* that day. My wife Val had done both, however. That evening she drew my attention to the letter. "Arn, she said, this might interest you." Val knew that while in practice at Simanowitz & Brown I had dealt with two medical negligence cases and had been shocked by both the treatment that the patients had received and the difficulties that I had encountered in trying to deal with the cases.

One of the cases I had dealt with was that of Dave Herriot. He had been a close friend of mine. A hard-drinking Irishman who, having left school without qualifications, had derived great benefit from studying at Ruskin College. He was tough as nails and a lovely man. In 1977 he went to Kenya on holiday, the first time he had been abroad. I did not see him on his return but phoned him shortly afterwards. He sounded rough. I asked him what was wrong. He said he felt awful and had been in bed for three days. In ten years I had never known Dave to take to his bed (at least not through illness!). Indeed if I ever complained of a cold he would accuse me of being a typical office-bound softie. (Not withstanding his education, Dave himself continued to work on a building site – in all weathers.)

He had actually been to see his GP for the first time. After a cursory examination he had diagnosed flu and told him to stay in bed. Three days later Dave was dead. He had had the most virulent form of malaria, plasmodium falciparum. He left a wife and two young daughters. Without any experience in medical negligence I advised his wife to consider making a claim for compensation. After all, Dave had come back from Kenya with a terrific tan in the middle of winter. Furthermore, he had never had to consult his doctor before. The GP had made no attempt to find out where Dave had been or to what he had been exposed. In a matter of minutes he had diagnosed flu. I obtained a short report from a GP. He stated that with the increased travel by British residents to more exotic destinations, and the increase of incidents of malaria, doctors had been advised for some time to look out for symptoms of that disease which could be mistaken for flu.

Armed with that I was able to obtain a Legal Aid certificate. The doctor's solicitors, appointed by his defence organisation, denied liability. They were able to exploit my inexperience and by 1982, when I finally stopped working at Simanowitz and Brown, the case was neither settled nor near trial. In fact it was not until some years later that the widow's new solicitors were able to negotiate a settlement in a very limited sum. Those solicitors too were inexperienced and did not have the courage or the knowledge to refuse an offer which was probably a quarter of what the widow and children were entitled to.

The other case was more bizarre. Mr Trotter had entered hospital for a liver operation. He died shortly after the operation. Although Mrs Trotter had no grounds for suspicion, she was very badly affected by the loss of her husband and she suspected that the doctors had poisoned him. I was referred the case by her daughter after three previous firms of solicitors had spent four years writing letters and getting nowhere. They had not even obtained an expert's opinion. Clearly there were unusual aspects to the treatment, and death after the type of operation Mr Trotter had undergone was most unusual.

By the time I was instructed, the limitation period had expired which meant that we were out of time to sue the hospital or the doctors involved. I had no alternative but to advise Mrs Trotter to take proceedings against the two firms of solicitors responsible for the delay which had led to any proceedings against the hospital or doctors being time-barred. Mrs Trotter was not very happy with this as she wanted those responsible for her husband's death to be sued. Her primary reason, however, for taking proceedings was to find out what had happened to her husband. I was therefore able to re-assure her that to succeed against the solicitors it would be necessary to prove that there had been a valid claim against the hospital or doctors which would mean a full examination of the cause of death and the responsibility for it.

Ironically it was easier to obtain a legal aid certificate for those proceedings than it would have been for the original claim. That was because the negligence of the solicitors was clear and it was causation, that is whether their delay had actually caused the damage, which would only become clear on examination of the medical issues.

Nevertheless I too was not able to progress the case, partly through my own lack of experience and partly because I was not able to find a liver specialist prepared to help. As a result the case dragged on in my hands as well and by the time I left Simanowitz and Brown it had still not been resolved. I had however become alive to the very real problems faced by those who, or whose loved ones, had suffered a medical accident.

I digress to tell an amusing story about Mrs Trotter but one which demonstrates the effect the loss of a loved one through a medical accident can have. I was attending a conference with a barrister with her when she suddenly mentioned that she had seen her husband. The barrister, without batting an eyelid, asked for details and she said she had seen him in the market a few days previously but before she could speak to him he had disappeared. The barrister, with an absolutely straight face explained to Mrs Trotter that it would be very difficult to pursue a claim for damages for the death of her husband if in fact he was still alive. She never mentioned her husband's appearance again.

As a result of my experience with these two cases I was certainly interested in following up Peter Ransley's letter. Indeed it immediately struck me that this might be the answer to the question I posed at the end of chapter one, "What Next?" Having disposed of Simanowitz & Brown I was looking for something community-based into which I could put my efforts. While looking around I was working as a locum at a South London firm of solicitors. I was determined to find something that satisfied my desire to do something for the community and to advance the cause of fairness and justice if only in a small way.

I wrote to Peter expressing my interest and telling him a bit of my background. He replied asking me to attend a preliminary meeting with other interested people to discuss the project. On the 1st February 1981 I turned up at the Ransley's door in Acton. Cynthia, Peter's wife opened the door. Upon announcing my name I noticed that she looked at me somewhat quizzically. She later told me that she had been surprised to see such a young man

(I was 43) as she had assumed from what I had said in my letter that I was a retired solicitor.

Gathered round the Ransley's kitchen table were the twelve people whom Peter and Cynthia had carefully selected from the large number who had responded to his letter. Peter and Cynthia, a medical social worker, were of course there. Then there was Stella Burnett herself. She was actually introduced to us as Kay Gilbert, the name given to her in the play. At that time she did not want her real identity disclosed for obvious reasons. The others were Marcia Saunders a secretary of a Community Health Council, Alan Edwards, a senior partner in the solicitors' firm of Douglas Mann & Co., whom Peter had known before, Helene Graham vice-Chair of a CHC, Tom Kerrane a Chief Nursing Officer, Clodagh Wilkinson a former member of a Regional Health Authority, Mary Sikkin and Dr Anne Savage a GP.

Not all of these remained involved. Three others joined the group some time later – Gwen Farrow a nurse journalist and her husband Derek Kartun, also a journalist, and Michael Ashby a Consultant neurologist. A decision having been taken to set up an organisation to help victims of medical accidents, the steering group eventually comprised Peter, Cynthia, Stella, Alan, Marcia, Michael, Gwen, Derek and me. I became secretary of the group and Alan agreed to look after any money we might receive.

We set about trying to attract funds, as we knew that to achieve anything a fairly substantial amount of money would be required. An obvious organisation to approach was The Kings Fund. After some correspondence we were invited to meet Robert Maxwell, the Chief Executive. Peter and I turned up at their rather sumptuous offices in Mornington Crescent where we were given tea and cucumber sandwiches. Sadly that was all we did receive from the Kings Fund at that time. Notwithstanding what I thought was a clear exposition of our aims, it was obvious that they thought we might turn out simply to be doctor bashers, and being one of the leading health charities they could not afford to be seen supporting something of that nature.

Applications to a number of other funds were also turned down. Our last hope was the Greater London Council. They were known to encourage more radical, less popular organisations that other more establishment funding organisations would not touch. I thought it might help too that I knew the Chair of ILEA (Inner

London Education Authority) who had started his political career in the seventies as a councillor in the London Borough of Croydon where I too had been a councillor.

This time it was Peter and Alan who went to the meeting with the GLC. They appeared to have a good reception. In subsequent conversations with my contact on the Council it all seemed very hopeful. So we began to gear up for a public launch. We had decided on the name Action for the Victims of Medical Accidents at the very first meeting of the Steering Group. There had been considerable discussion about this, particularly as we felt that the words "action" and "victim" could well be seen as provocative to the medical profession. In the end however, we all agreed that those two words were key as they encapsulated exactly what we were about and they indicated to patients whose side we were on.

We also had a logo – AVMA – and a letterhead. These had been designed by an advertising designer friend of Peter's, John Barlow. John later won an award for the design. I was particularly satisfied with the bold red colour of the design as it was not only striking but could also be interpreted to signify the blood that was often associated with medical procedures that went wrong. In addition we had someone to run the organisation. The Steering Committee had decided to offer me the job of Director in the event of our getting the grant. Perhaps they should have gone for open competition. That would certainly have been more in accordance with equal opportunities as currently understood. Bear in mind, however, that it was 1982 and most people's minds were not as focussed on the details of equal opportunities as they are today.

It was a bit tricky preparing for the launch because if we did not get the GLC grant it would have been rather a damp squib without funds to do anything. In fact, for the past year we had been struggling because people were still contacting Peter with their problems. While he now passed these on to me and I had a little more grasp of the issues – legal if not medical – there was not a lot we could do without any resources. The problem with the decision on the launch was that the BBC had decided to repeat Minor Complications on BBC2 on the 3rd August 1982 and we considered that for maximum impact and publicity the launch should take place shortly before that. We would not learn about the decision on the GLC grant, however, until the 22nd July.

We decided that we had no alternative but to proceed with the launch on the 28th July. The venue was booked – The Press Centre, New Square, near Fleet Street (at the time still the centre of the English press); invitations to the media were sent out together with our first press release. This was an enormous risk. Even with limited publicity we anticipated a considerable response and I clearly would not have been able to take on a full-time position as Director without funds for a salary. Notwithstanding this, our press release was drafted on the basis that I would be the Director. This was not the last time that AVMA had to take a risk.

On the 22nd July I duly contacted the GLC and was informed that we had been awarded a grant of £25,000 for 18 months. Whilst this was incredibly exciting and caused great jubilation when it was reported to the Committee at its meeting later that day, for me it posed a considerable dilemma. I had already agreed to accept a limited salary on the basis of the budget we had submitted to the GLC. I was now being offered only 18 months' security. Against that I had been offered a partnership in the firm for which I had been working for the previous six months which I greatly admired both because of their radical philosophy and their professionalism. Could I afford to give up that security on the basis of an 18 month grant?

In the end it was no contest. Not only was this work that would fulfil the ambitions I had been nursing for so many years, but I had been immersed for the past year in the stories of many victims of medical accidents and the hardship and injustice they had had to suffer. I could not now let them and myself down. And so I accepted the position. (Years later Cynthia Ransley, with whom among others I had shared my dilemma, told me that she believed that had I opted for the security of the partnership I would not have been the sort of person they wanted for the job anyway!)

It is interesting to reflect on the fact that the GLC had given us a grant. This was the time when the GLC and Ken Livingstone, "Red Ken" were being highly criticised for some of the organisations which they funded. In fact there are many worthwhile organisations – some even considered mainstream today – which would never have got off the ground were it not for the GLC. AVMA is certainly one of those. Had the GLC not given us the funds it is highly unlikely that anyone else would have done. Victims of medical accidents, like many other minorities, owe a great deal to the foresight of the GLC.

The press release could now go out. It is interesting to reflect, in the light of what AVMA has achieved, on what we stated as our aims namely:

### Information
There is a need for much more specific information for people who have medical accidents.

### Statistics
There should be standard procedures for reporting 'untoward incidents'. We will press for central collection and public access to this kind of information.

### Out-of-court settlements
It would assist claimants to know previous settlements and these should be published.

### Publicity
AVMA will attempt to put these cases in context, and give medical accident victims as a whole a voice.

But it is what was expressed as "AVMA's ultimate aim" which set the parameters of AVMA's work and is as much applicable today as it was then – "To increase awareness of the problem both among the general public and within the medical profession. We do not seek to promote unnecessary litigation, but to make it easier for ordinary people to perceive and pursue necessary litigation to which they have a right. We are acutely aware and sympathetic to the problems of doctors and nurses and believe a more open attitude would, in the end, benefit them as well as the small minority who suffer medical accidents."

And so, on the 28th July 1982 AVMA was launched at a press conference. The conference was reasonably well attended and in addition to reports in many newspapers we were invited to send someone to appear on ITV News. Alan Edwards had warned me in the run-up to the launch that as Director I would have to do most of the public appearances. This was not something I had done before and when I went along to the ITV studios in Euston

Road I was absolutely terrified. My state was not improved by the fact that I had to wait and see on the TV monitor in the waiting room all the earlier items (and the advertisements) being dealt with. I was anxious to get it over with but the time seemed to drag on forever. I kept looking at my watch and I suddenly realised that the programme was nearing its end and I had still not been called. Just before it did end someone came out and said they were sorry but that there had been a crisis at the GLC and they had done an extended interview with Ken Livingstone and there was no time to do my interview. What an anti-climax! Despite the fact that Ken had been responsible for our grant, at that moment. I could have throttled him. Now I would have to go through first-time nerves all over again if I were called upon to do an interview in the future.

The GLC grant was £25,000 for 18 months, under £17,000 for a year. It covered only my salary and provision for office rent. I had agreed to accept £11,000 p.a. which was the figure we had put in our grant application. That left about £5,500 to cover the rent and furniture, equipment and stationery. No money had been awarded for a secretary. While I was on my own there was little point in obtaining premises. I could work from home. The organisation had been publicly launched (with my home telephone number as the contact point!) so we had to start operating. I had a small spare room in my house in South East London and I set it up as an office. I bought an answerphone. I already owned a second-hand typewriter. And we were off!

Those first months were, like my entire time at AVMA, exciting, challenging and frustrating. In the first month I received about five hundred letters from people who believed that they had been a victim of a medical accident. In addition the phone never stopped ringing. I would leave my office – perhaps to go to a local photocopy shop as I had no photocopier – and return an hour later to find twenty messages on the answerphone. While almost all the stories were heartbreaking, there were many for whom I could do nothing. One woman began to phone me at all hours of the day and night. She was obviously mentally disturbed. She may well have suffered a medical accident but I found it quite impossible to identify exactly what she was complaining about. I had to tell her that I couldn't help her. That did not stop her and she continued to phone regularly, irrespective of the time. I could immediately recognise who it was because she always began her conversation in a hesitating and somewhat whining voice by asking, "Is that AMVA?"

I came to dread her calls, partly I think because of my inability to offer her any help. Val began to dread the calls as well because we had a phone by the bed and calls at three o'clock in the morning were not a little disturbing. Each time I told the woman that I could not help her she seemed to accept it. Then there would be another call. Eventually I had to be firm. The phone rang at 2 a.m. "Is that AMVA?" I felt like saying no. Instead I said in a very angry tone that I had told her a number of times that I could not help her and I did not want to hear from her again and if I did I would simply put the receiver down. She rang off. Two minutes later the phone rang again. "I don't want to hear from you ever again," she said and banged down the phone. Fortunately (for me) I never did hear from her again.

Some of the other calls and letters were from people who had been suffering for anything up to 30 years. One letter was from the father of a young man who had been a lad of 16 in the mid-nineteen seventies. I shall call him John. He was playing football when he fell and hurt his arm. By the end of the game his wrist was in agony. His parents took him to accident and emergency where a fracture of one the small bones in the wrist was diagnosed. His wrist was put in plaster and he was sent home. Because the small wrist bones can take a long time to heal he was told to return in six weeks.

After six weeks an X-ray showed that the bone had still not healed. New plaster was applied and remained on for another six weeks. Happily by then the bone had healed perfectly. It soon became apparent, however, that John had restricted use of his wrist. He returned to the hospital with his parents. The consultant explained that because of the length of time in plaster the wrist had developed adhesions – bands of fibrous tissue which join parts of the bone and can restrict movement. The solution was to manipulate the wrist under general anaesthetic which would break the adhesions. The consultant told the parents that he happened to have a vacancy the following week when he could perform the operation.

His parents wanted their son's problem to be dealt with as soon as possible but told the surgeon that unfortunately they had made arrangements to go to Paris for a week and as John was only 16 years old they would want to be present when the procedure was carried out. The consultant explained that the procedure was a routine one and although a general anaesthetic was involved it really was a simple matter and John would be home the same day. There was absolutely no need for them to be present. Totally reassured, the parents agreed to the early admission and when the time came happily set off for Paris.

While they were away John underwent the operation. When he woke up he was, surprisingly, in a private ward with nobody around. Still suffering the effects of the anaesthetic, he gradually became more aware of his surroundings. His injured arm began to itch and he lifted up the bedclothes to scratch it and discovered – that the arm had gone. The parents returned from Paris in due course and were horrified to discover what had happened.

But there was more to come. The parents were devastated. They wanted to know what had happened and how. At first they did not even think of compensation. The media and some of the medical profession would have us think that the first thought that comes into the minds of those who have suffered a medical accident or of their families, is "what can we get for it?" Even today, with all the hype about the compensation culture, that is not the case. There is no doubt, however, that at the time of this accident it was rare indeed for people to think of claims against health carers.

The parents approached the hospital. Initially they could get no explanation. After numerous frustrating telephone calls and meetings, as well as lengthy correspondence, gradually going higher up the chain of command in the hospital, they were eventually simply told that there had been a "mix up" with patients, resulting in their son having the wrong operation. No further explanation, no apology, no offer of compensation. No suggestion that the hospital would be taking steps to ensure that something like that could not happen again. Apparently no thought either about John's future problems and needs which would require considerable financial support if he were to come anywhere near to leading a normal life with his disability. The parents felt wholly frustrated, and deeply concerned about the nature of the damage. Unlike the health service carers they were acutely aware of the extreme disability with which their son would be left for the rest of his life. They were also by now angry not only about what had happened but also about the way they and their son had been treated following the accident.

They therefore consulted solicitors. They were persuaded that the only way they would get a proper response would be by seeking compensation. After about a year the hospital made an offer of substantial compensation. But the hospital not only did not admit negligence but actually made it a condition of the payment that nobody should be told about the incident or the payment.

The parents (and their solicitor) regarded the attaching of a "gagging clause" to the offer of settlement as tantamount to blackmail but they had no alternative but to accept it as the sum they were offered was greater than that which they would have been awarded had they litigated and was available without the tortuous, uncertain and lengthy process of litigation. I leave it to the reader to decide why the hospital was so generous.

When the boy's father wrote to me he enclosed a lovely photo of his son, now grown up, playing football with his own small son, the stump of the arm waving in the air. As can be imagined I was horrified by the story. I wanted to expose what had happened. I asked the father for permission to do so. He pointed out that he was bound by the settlement not to tell anyone about it and was even worried that he had told me.

I wrote and explained to him that I was satisfied that that agreement was unenforceable and even if it were enforceable the hospital would be far too ashamed to try and enforce it. I never heard from him again. What seemed so awful was that not only did the health carers ignore the fact that it was possible that something had gone wrong, but according to the clients, they did not appear to be prepared to do anything about the condition with which their patient had been left. It seemed to me that their GP (and often it is the GP who could explain what had happened and not those responsible for the original care which might have gone wrong) was not prepared to address the problem in case in some way that suggested that something had in fact gone wrong with the original care.

Among the many people who approached me in the early days, in some ways the "AMVA" lady was one of the easier clients because it was clear that we could not help her. With those I felt did need investigation it was more difficult. Of course I knew what had to be done. The medical information needed to be analysed carefully and if the treatment did appear to have been substandard and negligent then an experienced solicitor needed to make a claim on behalf of the client. But who was going to make a fair medical analysis and where were the experienced solicitors? As far as preliminary medical analysis was concerned, all I could do in those first days was to ask the doctor on AVMA's committee to give a preliminary opinion. However, I had also learned from Peter Ransley's play that it was possible for a lay person, with the help of medical books, to go some way towards at least understanding the logic of a medical opinion.

John's case, and that of Stella Burnett, encapsulates the situation that pertained thirty years ago when things went wrong during medical care. The underlying culture, which the public was encouraged to accept, was that mistakes did not happen. As a result no explanations were voluntarily tendered even when the most disastrous consequences ensued, and if anyone had the temerity to enquire what had gone wrong they were met with obstruction, denial and cover-up. Unless of course the mistake was so obvious that it could not be hidden, as in John's case.

The problem was that there was no one who understood the system well enough to be able to make pertinent enquiries and who would not blindly accept explanations tendered by the healthcare professionals. In John's case the hospital was so determined that nobody should be able to learn that mistakes did happen that they were prepared to pay over the odds in order to try to ensure that the settlement was never reported. The solicitor happily advised his clients to accept that situation without realising that it was an immoral condition and even if imposed could not be enforced. Imagine if, having accepted the compensation, the parents had gone public. Would the hospital have courted further adverse publicity by demanding repayment of the money, even if such a condition had been enforceable?

In my opinion, however, that was not the most important issue. It may well be that healthcare professionals felt safe from exposure because no one was really able to challenge them effectively. But what about the Hippocratic Oath? What about the wider responsibility of the National Health Service to its patients and their relatives? And what about the fundamental question of patient safety?

Why was it possible that the members of what is arguably the most caring of professions did not want to explain what had happened and try to alleviate the consequences, if necessary by ensuring that the injured patient received sufficient compensation to restore at least some of their lost quality of life? Could those working for the NHS really believe that after an accident in the course of medical care they had no responsibility to the patient and his or her family? And why did nobody in the NHS or indeed the medical profession realise that by covering up every adverse incident (as medical accidents have now come to be called) they were denying the opportunity of all others working in the NHS to learn from mistakes?

Of course, the issue of compensation was an important one particularly for those whose quality of life had been substantially affected by the negligent acts of healthcare professionals. Indeed, in the absence of a sudden change in the prevailing culture and attitudes of the healthcare professionals, it would only be by improving the way in which medical negligence litigation was conducted that patients who had been harmed during medical care would have a chance of receiving the compensation to which they were entitled and perhaps an investigation into the causes of the accident. So I shall look first at the issue of compensation but in due course will try to address some of the wider questions I have raised.

# Chapter 3
# Medical negligence

I shall deal with the law relating to medical negligence (now known as clinical negligence) in a later chapter (see chapter 7) but as the word negligence has already cropped up and will be repeatedly used throughout the book it is as well that I define it at this stage. That is particularly important for those reading this book who have no knowledge of the subject.

I can best define negligence, and indeed medical negligence, by quoting the words of the judge in the seminal medical negligence case of *Bolam v Friern Hospital Management Committee 1957 Queens Bench Division*:

> "In the ordinary case which does not involve any special skill, negligence in law means this: Some failure to do some act which a reasonable man in the circumstances would do, or doing some act which a reasonable man in the circumstances would not do; and if that failure or doing of that act results in injury, then there is a cause of action. How do you test whether this act or failure is negligent? In an ordinary case it is generally said that you judge that by the action of the man in the street. He is the ordinary man. In one case it has been said that you judge it by the conduct of the man on the top of a Clapham Omnibus. He is the ordinary man.
>
> But where you get a situation which involves the use of some special skill or competence, then the test whether there has been negligence or not is not the test of the man on the top of a Clapham Omnibus because he has not got this special skill. The test is the standard of the ordinary skilled man exercising and professing to have that special skill. A man need not possess the highest skill at the risk of being found negligent. It is well established law that it is

sufficient if he exercises the ordinary skill of an ordinary competent man exercising that particular art."

But who says whether he was exercising that ordinary skill? The judgement went on to say that "A doctor is not guilty of negligence if he acted in accordance with a practice accepted as proper by a responsible body of medical men skilled in that particular art". Reduced to its simplest, what that amounts to is that if a number of experienced medical people, that is, "a responsible body", say that the action of the doctor was reasonable then the doctor is not negligent. That definition, modified only slightly as explained below has bedevilled the ability of victims of a medical accident to obtain compensation.

I would add two things in connection with that definition. Firstly I suspect that today the definition might also refer to the "reasonable woman". Secondly, the definition was slightly refined in 1997 in the case of *Bolitho v City and Hackney Health Authority*. In that case it was held that "the court should not accept a defence argument as being 'reasonable', 'respectable' or 'responsible' without first assessing whether such opinion is susceptible to logical analysis".

I would suggest that any reasonable person, looking at this definition, would think that this is a clear case of the professions looking after their own. In all other situations it is the Judge who decides whether someone has been reasonable. In the case of doctors it appears that Judges are saying let the medical profession itself decide. Of course, in practice, the Judges do make the decision, and the decision in the case of *Bolitho* has made it easier for them to break away from the opinion of "a responsible body of medical men." They do that in many cases by "preferring" the evidence of the claimant's medical experts (a responsible body) to that of the defendant's medical experts (also a responsible body). Nevertheless it is quite clear that because of the definition, it is the medical profession, one of whose members is in trouble, that has control of the case.

So let us look at the state of medical negligence litigation at the time of the cases in the previous chapter, which might explain why Stella Burnett and John were treated as they were.

If you are going to embark on legal proceedings it is wise to engage a solicitor who is experienced in the type of litigation involved. This is even more important where there is a lot at stake and you are challenging one of the most powerful institutions. In that situation nothing less than an expert in the area will do. In the seventies medical negligence litigation was not a recognised expertise. Of course there were a few solicitors who had some experience in this litigation. But unlike many other areas of the law there was no knowledgeable pool of medical negligence solicitors. This was due to the existence of a Catch 22.

This catch began with the idea that litigation against the medical profession was difficult if not impossible. As a result any solicitor approached to take on such a case would shake his head, suck in his breath and indicate that it was inadvisable. "It would cost an arm and a leg", he would say, and it would be impossible to prove negligence against a doctor whose profession would back him to the hilt. So solicitors would not take on cases. Consequently they could not gain the experience to become expert. And not having the expertise they would continue to believe that such cases were hopeless and therefore refuse to take on these cases.

The doctors' solicitors were, however, in a totally different position. In England and Northern Ireland (Scotland operates under a different legal system, though the results are not dissimilar) there were two firms who specialised in undertaking the defence of doctors. They were the firms that acted for the two organisations which advised doctors who were in trouble, the Medical Protection Society and the Medical Defence Union. Together they covered virtually all the cases that were brought against doctors individually. The amount of litigation that was taking place at that time can be seen from the number of Legal Aid Certificates that were issued for such cases. As I will explain later the vast majority of such cases would need to be supported by legal aid. In 1981 only 800 certificates were issued. If that number were divided equally between the two defence firms that would mean that each was dealing with 400 cases a year. Clearly the division would not have been so precise but each firm must have at least been dealing with over 200 cases each year — sufficient to become highly expert.

Divide those cases among the thousands of solicitors dealing with litigation generally however, or even personal injury cases specifically, and it is clear that it would be rare for a claimant's solicitor to see more than one case a year. As a result, in those cases that were commenced, the defence solicitors could generally run rings around the claimant's solicitors – which of course discouraged any solicitor from taking on any further cases.

The suggestion that a medical negligence case would "cost an arm and a leg" was also true at that time. That only 800 Legal Aid certificates were issued in 1981 was not simply due to the fact that only a small number of certificates were applied for. There was also the fact that the solicitors did not submit any evidence to the Law Society (which was the body that at that time dealt with legal aid applications) to enable their administrators looking at the application to judge whether there was a good case or not. To some extent it was not the fault of the solicitors that they did not submit any evidence with their application. It was not at that time the practice of the Law Society to issue a Legal Aid certificate limited to obtaining a medical report, so usually solicitors had no funds to obtain medical evidence. The administrators of the Legal Aid scheme then, instead of suggesting to the solicitor that he or she should seek some medical evidence or, indeed, issuing a certificate limited to obtaining such evidence, would simply judge on what they saw before them. Given the prevailing attitude that doctors were never negligent, engendered and cultivated by the profession itself and compounded by the deference shown to doctors generally, it was not surprising that most applications were refused off the cuff, as it were. So that was the second limb of the Catch 22 – you can't get a Legal Aid certificate without the medical evidence, but you can't get the medical evidence without a Legal Aid certificate.

If Legal Aid was refused then the only recourse for the patient was to fund the case privately. The work involved in preparing a medical negligence case properly was considerable. The medical records had to be obtained, a medical expert instructed, Counsel instructed to draft the pleadings and research carried out. The trial itself might last two weeks or more. The costs in those days might be anything from £10,000 to £100,000. Furthermore, if the patient lost the case they would be ordered by the court to pay the defendant's costs. They could be looking at a final bill of £200,000. "An arm and a leg" was right. No ordinary person could contemplate such expenditure. And at that time it was against the law to undertake the case speculatively, that is on the basis that the client would only pay if the case were won.

There must be many patients who were seriously injured by the grossest negligence in the past who continue to suffer today without having received compensation. Indeed even today solicitors are commencing, and winning, cases where the injury occurred anything up to 30 years ago.

One of the reasons why solicitors did not have success either with their Legal Aid applications or with the cases themselves was their belief that medical negligence litigation was the same as personal injury litigation. Personal injury relates to harm caused to individuals in an accident. Clearly someone who was hurt in a medical accident had suffered a personal injury. Even in personal injury litigation there were many solicitors who had the wrong approach, hence the need for the establishment of the Association of Personal Injury Lawyers (APIL) in 1990 which is dealt with in chapter 5. However, even the solicitors who were proficient in personal injury litigation had problems with medical negligence litigation because they believed it could be approached in the same way. After all, they were dealing with a client who had suffered a personal injury so why not?

But there were major differences. When an "ordinary" accident takes place even lay people can see that there may be a dispute as to who was at fault notwithstanding that it may not be an open and shut case. An official at the Law Society dealing with an application for legal aid was able to see, possibly with the assistance of a statement by a witness, that there would be a likelihood of success and would be prepared to issue a certificate. In the case of medical negligence however, it is rare to be able to see that there is a case of negligence in the absence of a medical expert's opinion. Therefore an application submitted without a medical report is almost bound to fail.

Furthermore, in seeking a medical expert's report there are two prerequisites in medical negligence litigation which do not apply in personal injury litigation. Firstly the expert must be one who is prepared to adopt an entirely objective approach and fearlessly to criticise his or her colleagues if necessary. At that time, when a solicitor did go to the trouble of instructing a medical expert, it was more often than not their friendly doctor who had helped them in numerous personal injury actions which did not involve criticising a colleague. That expert would invariably decide that no negligence was involved. To be fair, many of those doctors, who were inexperienced in dealing with medical negligence cases, did not really understand what was expected of them and were not told what was expected by their instructing solicitor who was probably as ignorant of that as was the doctor.

That leads to the second prerequisite in instructing an expert. The expert must be fully instructed. That means that the solicitor himself, or herself, must understand and get to grips with the medical issues involved in order both to be able to identify for the expert the questions that require answering, as well as to determine the quality of the report when it is received. To return to the case of Stella Burnett related at the beginning of the book: It was only because she carried out her own research and became fully aware of the medical issues involved, that she was able to identify the fact that her first expert had not addressed the issues and that her second expert was in fact suggesting that there had been negligence, although he did not say so in so many words. If a lay person was able to understand sufficient of the medical issues to identify these matters it is obvious that solicitors could do the same.

This was not as necessary in relation to ordinary personal injury litigation. Firstly the medical issues were not at the heart of the question as to whether negligence had occurred. Secondly, as a medical expert was only being employed to indicate the nature of the injuries and was not concerned with who the defendant was, it was more likely that he would give an objective report.

Unfortunately, at that time there were few solicitors who were able, or prepared, to get to grips with the medical issues even in the simplest case.

The problem of experts arriving at decisions on negligence in a somewhat cursory fashion was compounded by the fact that many experts either prepared their reports without recourse to the patient's medical records or refused to do the report without sight of the records which could not, in those days, be obtained easily or at all. Like the issue of the dearth of solicitors experienced in medical negligence litigation, the question of obtaining the medical records was also subject to a Catch 22. Until 1985, the only way records could be obtained was by a procedure for disclosure of documents which the courts allowed during the conduct of the litigation. In order to use that procedure, however, the litigation had to be in progress. In order to be able to obtain an expert's report which would justify the start of litigation the medical records were required. And they could not be obtained by court order because the litigation was not in progress.

Of course, the solicitors acting for the doctor, the hospital or the Health Authority could agree to the disclosure of the records but knowing that a court could not force them to do so they invariably refused, notwithstanding that they might know that the patient would thereby suffer injustice. This simple statement hides two further major problems that existed in this litigation at that time. The first involved the question of whom to sue. I have referred to the solicitors of the doctor, the hospital or the Health Authority. At that time each was treated as a separate entity and any one or all of them might be guilty of negligence. It was therefore necessary in many cases to name the doctor as well as the Health Authority because if the wrong defendant were sued the case could fail on that technicality rather than on the facts. Many solicitors were not aware of this problem and got themselves and their clients into serious difficulty.

This problem of acquiring the records in order to decide whether a case was likely to be successful was not solved until the case of *Hall v Wandsworth Health Authority [1985] 129 Sol Jo 188, 16 February* (discussed in Chapter 7).

Another problem that stood in the way of a victim of a medical accident securing compensation was even more fundamental, and to some extent still exists today. It relates to the way in which the medical profession and healthcare professionals generally viewed a medical accident and the patients who had suffered. It might be thought that when something went wrong in medical care the doctors would have gone to the furthest lengths to try and do something about it. After all, until something went wrong their calling, and indeed the Hippocratic Oath, impelled them to strive to do the best for their patient. Doctors in the UK do not now take any oath but are bound both by the ethical principles laid down in the oath promulgated by Hippocrates in the 5th century BCE, and the provisions of the doctors' "bible" *Good Medical Practice*. The clearest statement in the original oath with regard to patients, which still prevails today is that "I will keep them from harm and injustice".

Surely when a patient had suffered additionally as a result of a mistake the doctors would have tried even harder to care for the patient? In fact, what used to happen, and with some doctors it still happens today, was that the doctor would suddenly view the patient as a threat: someone who might damage their reputation or cost them money. The whole profession went into cover-up mode. It was impossible to get any information about what had happened and if legal proceedings were threatened or started the only concern on the part of the health-care professionals was to defeat the claim, irrespective of its merits. Indeed, often the patient did not receive any additional treatment required lest that be seen as an acknowledgement that something had in fact gone wrong.

No apology or explanation was forthcoming from a clinician or administrator. That was viewed as an admission of liability and an invitation to make a claim. Indeed if the patient did think that something had gone wrong and made a complaint the response would invariably be an outright denial. Alternatively, ambiguous wording would often be used to confuse the naïve patient. The most common example was "I am sorry you feel that you have been mistreated."

The charitable explanation for this behaviour, and indeed an understandable one, is that when a doctor does injure a patient he or she will be in denial. To injure your own patient, particularly if the injury is major, such as causing a baby to be brain-damaged, can be hugely traumatic, and extremely difficult to face. With such denial it is the arrival of the letter of claim or the beginning of legal proceedings which makes the doctor realise that his or her negligence may have been the cause.

The next problem for victims that pertained at that time is connected to that attitude of the medical profession. To some extent solicitors could not be blamed for not using the right kind of experts. In those days there were very few doctors prepared to act as experts in medical negligence litigation. On the one hand they were reluctant personally to criticise their colleagues. On the other hand the profession as a whole considered that any doctor who did give evidence for an injured patient was "letting down the side". In this connection, I was told a story by a consultant obstetrician who was one of the rare breed who was prepared to stick his neck out in those days. At a meeting of his college he overheard a senior member of that college telling a young doctor that if he gave evidence for patients against doctors "it would not do his career any good". So the conspiracy of silence that operated to ensure that doctors did not discuss their own or their colleagues' mistakes also meant that doctors were reluctant to act as experts on behalf of injured patients.

All these problems were serious obstacles in the way of patients securing their just compensation. However, the most important obstacle was in fact the way in which the legal procedure in these cases operated. From the beginning the dice were loaded against the claimant. When a claimant's lawyer instituted proceedings for compensation in the Court he or she had to set out in detail the nature of the claim and the facts on which the allegation of negligence was based, called in those days the Statement of Claim. These details would be based on the expert's report and would relate in great detail exactly what it was alleged had happened and why it was alleged that that amounted to negligence on the part of the defendant. I can recall at least one case in which the Statement of Claim ran to twenty-five pages.

Accordingly the defendant's solicitor knew precisely what claim the defendant had to meet. The defendant's solicitor then had to put in the defence. All that was required of the defendant in those days, however, was to deny the facts (if they were disputed) and/or to deny the negligence. A defence might be, and usually was, no more than one page. This situation was compounded by the fact that there was no requirement for the parties to exchange their expert reports. As a result the claimant would have absolutely no idea what the defendant was saying had actually happened and why he or she was denying negligence. This situation would pertain right up until the trial.

The first time the claimant's lawyers would begin to learn what the defendant's case was would be when the plaintiff's expert witness was being cross-examined. The detail of that case would only finally appear when the defendant's expert gave evidence. This meant that before the trial the defendant's lawyers could put the claimant's case to their client and to their expert witness. Their client could explain the discrepancies and the expert could, if necessary, carry out the necessary research to refute the claimant's medical case. I could not possibly suggest that in some cases experts could actually construct their report to meet the plaintiff's case but it did often look that way. The claimant's lawyer and expert had no such opportunity.

This procedure was described by many as trial by ambush. It is a clear indication of how the defence regarded the proceedings simply as a game. There were many cases in which, the claimant's expert hearing the defendant's case for the first time, and hearing the explanation of the defendant and evidence of the defence expert for the first time, he would concede that there was no negligence or a possibility that there was no negligence. The claimant's case would then collapse. Had the defendant's solicitor put that case to the claimant's solicitor at the outset there would have been a considerable saving of time and costs, both to the NHS and to the Legal Aid fund. The patient would also not have had the additional suffering of preparing for a court case on top of the suffering from the injury which had been caused. Nor would she or he have had their expectation of much-needed compensation raised unnecessarily. Instead of having their whole life tied up with dealing with the case over a number of years they would have been able to concentrate on accepting the situation and rebuilding their lives. All of this did not appear to have been any concern of the doctors, their defence organisations, the hospital authorities or the defence solicitors. When addressing audiences of health providers as I came to do, I made this point repeatedly but it was many years before it made any impression at all.

Of course it suited the defendants, if they had no concern for the suffering of the patient or relatives, to maintain this situation of ambush. No better example of this determination to keep the claimant in the dark can be seen than in the case of *Hall v Wandsworth Health Authority* to which I have already referred, where the defendants resisted disclosure of the medical records before the claimant had issued proceedings even though they knew that those records would demonstrate to the claimant that there had been no negligence. I deal with that case in more detail in chapter 6.

I have referred to a claimant's life being tied up for a number of years while pursuing a claim. Those solicitors dealing with clinical negligence litigation today who have only in recent years entered this field might be surprised at just how long most cases used to take. This was caused by a combination of three things.

Firstly the tactics of the defendants. From the resistance to the disclosure of records, through the failure to divulge information and the taking of every possible technical point against the claimants, good or bad, to the delay in dealing with the pleadings, the defendants' solicitors adopted every delaying tactic they could in the hope that the claimants or their solicitors would despair or run out of funds.

The second cause of delay was the inexperience of the claimants' solicitors. Not only were they unable to deal adequately with the defendants' solicitors' delaying tactics but they were themselves unable to progress the case for long periods simply because they did not know what to do. And finally there was no oversight by the Court of the progress of the case. The litigants were simply left to get on with the case or not. The result was that the majority of cases would drag on for anything up to ten years. Indeed some cases were a challenge to the record held by *Jarndyce vs Jarndyce* in *Bleak House*.

# Chapter 4
# Progress

By doing my own research and reading up on the medical issues which began to present themselves with increasing repetition, I began to see that even the well-meaning and sympathetic doctor who had later joined the committee was so steeped in the medical culture that his opinions were based on the assumption that the medical team concerned had probably done the right thing. In the cases where, either because of our doctor's opinion or more frequently despite it, I formed the view that a case was worth investigating the next question was to which solicitors I could refer them. For the reasons I explained in chapter 3 I was not aware of any solicitors who were expert in medical negligence. I decided to start with solicitors whom I knew personally and whom I considered to be highly competent in personal injury litigation. I could discuss the cases with them and together we could learn about the nuances in medical negligence. They had the further advantage of having good relationships with a number of medical experts whom they used in "ordinary" personal injury cases. They were able to persuade a few of them to assist in their medical negligence cases and to impress on them what was needed in such cases.

Of course all of us were only beginning to learn about what was virtually a new branch of the law. I have no doubt that in those early days we accepted negative opinions from some experts who were not sufficiently rigorous. Under knowledgeable scrutiny by a solicitor or by me it might have been possible to recognise the flaws and pursue the case further. It still bothers me that in those days people with potentially good cases may have been discouraged from seeking compensation by those upon whom they and we were relying.

It was not only the cases of those who had been injured, or believed themselves to have been injured, in a medical accident which I had to tackle. There was also the major issue of how to bring about change in the way the issue of medical accidents was approached – by the health carers, by the health administrators and by the government. At heart this was an issue of patient safety. Indeed, the most exciting thing about the challenge of the job I was facing was the fact that it was many-faceted.

It seemed to me that the first thing we had to do was to identify the size of the problem. It was clear even from the reaction we had had since our launch that there was quite a number of people who had suffered. That did not, however, tell us whether we were facing a problem involving hundreds a year, thousands or even millions. I immediately ran into a problem. There were no statistics in the UK. Of course that was not surprising because it had become abundantly clear that nobody recognised medical accidents as an issue that needed addressing. Even nearly two years after AVMA was started the implications of things going wrong were not realised. I commented on this in a letter to the BMJ in May 1984 (BMJ Volume 288 p1460) about the Confidential Enquiry into Peri-natal Deaths (CEPOD) in Wessex in 1981 and 1982. One of the statistics produced in the report of that inquiry showed that in the Wessex Regional Health Authority there were 5.8 neonatal deaths per 1000 live births that may have been contributed to by "adverse factors in medical care", in other words a medical accident. I wrote that I was able to extrapolate from that the possibility that in England alone there could be nearly 3000 neonatal deaths caused by adverse factors in medical care. That implication was either overlooked or discounted for certainly no action was taken to address it, even after my letter.

Neither were there any statistics elsewhere. The United States appeared to be the only country that was doing any work on the subject but it was not until some years later that research was published there that gave an inkling of the size of the problem in that country. For the time being we simply had to go on the fact that the number of people who were approaching us was increasing daily. That was despite the fact that, because I had to deal with everything myself, we were, apart from the publicity received at the time of the launch, not even advertising our existence.

We also had to address the issue of change. We recognised that although we were focussing on medical accidents, the main issue was in fact patient safety. Patient safety today is almost the watchword of the NHS and indeed a government body called the National Patient Safety Agency (NPSA) was established in 2001. The purpose of the NPSA was to collect information about all adverse incidents that occurred in NHS hospitals, and to feed this information back so that hospitals would be obliged to take steps to ensure that such incidents did not happen anywhere again. It was a measure of AVMA's achievement by that stage that I was appointed as a non-executive Director on that body. When AVMA started, however, the expression "Patient safety" was rarely if ever used. In fact, AVMA itself never used the term. Effectively, however, we were the first organisation to try to address patient safety. If due attention were paid to patients' safety that would automatically reduce the number of avoidable accidents. Or, to put it another way, if due attention were paid to reducing the number of avoidable accidents that would automatically increase patient safety. To achieve this there would have to be a change in the culture of healthcare professionals. At the same time there was a need to change the way victims of medical accidents could secure compensation. Although AVMA's *raison d'être* was not simply to increase and improve litigation and compensation, I believed that we would only begin to achieve both these changes if we did increase the number and success rate of claims against doctors and the Health Service. By hitting doctors where it hurt most, in their pockets, and by increasing the cost to the NHS, we would be bound to get some reaction.

Two comments by Dr Armond Gwynne of the Medical Defence Union in an article by Yvonne Roberts in *The Standard* (latterly the *Evening Standard*) on the 31st December 1982 demonstrated exactly why litigation would have to be the key. Firstly he complained that as a result of the "fourfold" increase in the number of cases of medical negligence in the past five years the annual fee to doctors for protection would be increased by 40% – to £195! (By contrast today there are varying rates of subscription, all in the thousands of pounds.) Secondly he argued that "the present system of compensation works fairly". Together those statements demonstrated a complacency about the problem which had to be challenged in the most drastic fashion.

We were, however, fully aware that it was necessary to take doctors with us. Unless we could do so, all our efforts would be sabotaged. After all, a culture cannot be changed without the co-operation of those whose culture is to be changed. How to pursue both these ends was the most formidable challenge facing us. With regard to the attitude of doctors, our greatest asset was the doctors themselves. After all, I liked to see the medical profession as the most caring of professions and I always referred to them as such. Most doctors entered the profession with the highest ideals. Their aim was to help people, to cure them, not to damage them. It was simply a question of tapping into those ideals in relation to the specific issues of safety and medical accidents.

After about six months working from the back room in my home I was able to find premises in Stockwell Road in Brixton. Why Brixton? Well, firstly at that stage I had the luxury of only having myself to please in terms of convenience. Brixton was only a short bus or car ride from my home in Upper Norwood. Of course I wanted the office to be as accessible to the public as possible so there was no question of setting up in Upper Norwood itself or its surrounds. Secondly, our budget for rent did not run to anything more central and those premises were really cheap. I did not realise at the time that one of the reasons for that was that they backed onto what was then the most notorious Council estate in Brixton. (The nature of the area was to be brought home to us later. Two members of our small staff suffered losses. On one occasion someone simply walked in off the street and stole a handbag lying on a desk. The other incident was more serious when our Deputy Director was mugged just outside the office and though not badly injured was very shaken. These incidents contributed to our decision to move from Brixton when we did.)

At the same time I had been able to secure a one-off grant from the Joseph Rowntree Charitable Trust to pay the salary of a secretary for a year. (Looking back it is hard to believe that £5,000 was enough to cover salary and all associated expenses but then I myself was only being paid £11,000 a year!) The receipt of the grant and the finding of the premises could not have been more timely. We were beginning to receive quite a lot of publicity. I had finally made my first TV appearance – fortunately not live. Channel 4 had commissioned a full-length documentary on the subject and the interviewer, Helena Kennedy (now Baroness) had had to interview me in my sitting room. That had generated a substantial response and I was beginning to find it impossible to cope on my own and the backlog was piling up. Ironically, that set the pattern for the future of AVMA. As the organisation expanded over the years we were never, during my time as Chief Executive, able to catch up with the backlog as the number of people approaching us increased and our resources never grew fast enough to keep pace.

Not all of the publicity we received was positive. *GP*, one of the medical free papers, contacted me as they were doing an article about AVMA and wanted a photograph of me. The photographer duly appeared at our premises in Stockwell Road. He cajoled me into going outside for the photo. I guess I was pretty naïve because he persuaded me that standing behind some building scaffolding would make a nice frame for the photo. When the article appeared, with my long hair and beard the photograph portrayed me as a wild man behind bars. Fortunately the article itself was sympathetic and gave publicity to the fact that in the year since we had been founded we had discovered something which is now universally accepted, save perhaps by a small number of doctors – that when something goes wrong in medical treatment "People clearly want to know what happened and why, and the desire for an apology is far greater than a wish for compensation." (*GP* 7th October 1983)

The process of recruiting a secretary threw an interesting light on how some lawyers operate. One of the solicitors who had been recommended to me by someone whose judgement I trusted was a top-class personal injury lawyer who acted for a number of Unions. I was beginning to refer a number of cases to him and clearly he wanted to break into this area. When I mentioned to him that I was looking for a secretary he told me that his wife was looking for a position. She was a brilliant secretary, he said, and would be ideal for this position. I told him that she would have to apply like everyone else which he appeared to accept. Not long after I was delighted to receive a donation to AVMA from him of £150 which was a lot of money in those days. In due course, because his wife was clearly well qualified I interviewed her along with a number of others.

Ultimately I decided that while she definitely had excellent secretarial skills I needed someone who had more commitment to the problems of medical accident victims and who could to some extent work in partnership with me given that she would for some time to come be the only other employee. She was clearly not in that category and I appointed another candidate, Wendy Gorst, who proved to be just what I had needed. When I told her husband he was absolutely furious and in his anger blurted out that he would not have sent me the £150 had he not expected his wife to be appointed.

This was a major lesson for me. As a solicitor myself, I knew that people went into the Law with mixed motives. Most believed that they would be providing a worthwhile service to society. At the same time they recognised that the law was a profession of high status and in most cases extremely well paid. In my view there were two other groups at either end of the spectrum. One comprised those who were only interested in the money and were not too bothered about ethics. With the others their main motivation was in fact to help those who had suffered in some way and could only be helped through the Law. They have a high moral and ethical sense. It is people of that ilk who end up working in civil liberties and the more social and less well paid end of the Law such as acting for tenants, refugees, charities and victims of domestic violence.

I do not want in any way to undervalue those who go in with mixed motives. Most of them do an excellent and essential job and do indeed perform a service for society. They are honest and hardworking whilst reaping a considerable reward. It was clear to me from the outset, however, and reinforced by this incident of the appointment of a secretary, that it was from the last-mentioned group that I wanted to recruit solicitors for medical negligence. We had a big battle ahead and there was no guarantee that the rewards would be great. Furthermore, we did not wish to be tarred with the brush of simply being about suing doctors for compensation. It was true that we would ourselves be devoting a large part of our work to campaigning for patient safety and for justice for victims of medical accidents. However, we would want the lawyers who acted for our clients also to be committed to these aims and supporting AVMA as well as securing maximum compensation for their clients. What we needed were first-rate lawyers who would be prepared to put their considerable skills towards achieving these objectives.

In the beginning finding such solicitors was somewhat hit and miss. I started working with solicitors I knew. Before the founding of AVMA I had been working as a locum at a firm in South London. This was the radical practice Fisher Meredith which handled a lot of personal injury cases including an occasional medical negligence case, some of which I had had to deal with during my locum. The partner whose work I had been doing as a locum while she was on maternity leave was Anne Winyard. I had great respect for her, having seen the impeccable way in which she had dealt with her cases and we had had many discussions about medical negligence. She was totally committed to the idea of helping victims and was well aware of the difficulties that were placed in the way of their achieving justice. I had no hesitation in recruiting her as my very first "referral" solicitor.

Because Anne worked in the field of personal injury she was able to recommend others in that field whom she considered to be highly competent solicitors who were absolutely committed to doing the best for their clients. In addition, as a result of the publicity I was contacted by others who expressed an interest in helping victims of medical accidents. One was Philip Sycamore, who later became a Circuit Judge. His practice was in Blackpool but he came all the way down to see me and we spent some time over coffee discussing the issues and the hurdles. Although I knew nothing of his track record it was clear that he had a great interest in the subject and would be totally committed to helping victims. Another solicitor who contacted me as a result of the publicity was David Body who later became one of the leading solicitors in medical negligence litigation. He was not even a personal injury specialist but it was clear from my conversation with him that he was both extremely clever and very keen to use his talents in the interests of victims.

In fact what I was doing was starting the beginning of a virtuous circle. In the same way as the vicious circle had operated, with solicitors not taking on medical negligence cases and therefore being inexperienced and consequently being unwilling to take on cases, I was now reversing the process. As AVMA referred more cases to the small band of solicitors whom I had gathered around me, so they became more experienced, more proficient and more successful – and of course, more keen to take on cases. However, what had become clear to me pretty soon after starting to work with AVMA was that the key to helping clients with their legal claims was understanding the medical issues. I couldn't even begin to decide whether to refer a case on to solicitors, or once having referred it on being able to see whether the case was being conducted properly, without that understanding. So instead of simply saying to myself when a client sent in information, I'll leave the medical issues to the medical experts, I began to read up on those issues. The solicitors to whom I was referring cases would have to do the same. After all, if Stella Burnett had been able to grasp medical issues, there did not appear to be any reason why we should not be able to do so.

Of course, it was more difficult for me as in most cases I would not have the medical records. Nevertheless, with a detailed statement from the client as to the condition she or he had been suffering from, the treatment that had been given, and the outcome, I could, by reading medical books and getting help from a friendly doctor, at least form a preliminary view of the situation. I could also begin to understand something of the human body. The availability of friendly doctors was absolutely crucial. It was not simply a question of having a doctor who would prepare an honest opinion when instructed and paid. What both I and the solicitors needed in those early days were doctors who believed in what we were doing and were prepared to spend time, free of charge, helping us and teaching us. I shall deal in greater detail with the whole issue of medical experts in a later chapter. However, at that time the identification of truly helpful doctors by both me and the solicitors I was working with was fundamental. It is a credit to those doctors who were prepared to help that they were prepared to risk the ire of their colleagues to help patients to litigate against some of those colleagues.

There were two consultant obstetricians like that who were already working in the field. The first was the late Professor Peter Huntingford. Patients owe a huge debt of gratitude to Peter. I was introduced to him early on and it was quite clear that he was convinced that it was the duty of the medical profession to help those who had been let down by that profession. He also believed that exposing the mistakes that doctors made would lead to better medicine as doctors learned from experience – a true early exponent of patient safety. Sadly by the time of his death in October 2000 that second belief had not been vindicated. The other doctor who was extremely helpful to me and the first solicitors in AVMA's team was Roger Clements. In addition, I received personal advice and assistance from my brother Milton, also a consultant obstetrician who became interested because of my involvement.

It is significant that all three were obstetricians: The consequences of mistakes in the delivery of a baby were invariably more disastrous than in most other areas of medicine. Brain-damaged babies were then, as now, the most heart-rending cases. In the main they also attract the largest awards of damages. That is because if a baby is damaged at birth in such a way that he or she will never be able to look after themselves, their care will be required for a lifetime. Round-the-clock care for that length of time is extremely costly. Obstetricians clearly were aware of the dangers and probably all of them knew that many of those disasters could have been avoided. In those early days it appeared that only doctors like those I have mentioned believed that parents were entitled to know the truth about what had happened and that the children were entitled to the lifelong support that only a successful legal claim could bring.

These doctors did attract the ire of their colleagues. They were considered to be letting down the side. The incident involving a consultant's advice to a more junior colleague which I described earlier where a Consultant warned a junior doctor against helping medical accident victims is one of the more blatant examples of this. However, some doctors reading about AVMA did react positively. One of the first of those to contact us was a Scottish surgeon, David Hamilton, who approached us in August 1982 offering to help. He was of great help in the early years, being prepared not only to act as an expert for patients but often helping me with informal advice. He was one of the first doctors to give me behind-the-scenes insights into how doctors themselves knew the risks of procedures which they did not pass on to their patients. For example, he told me that in the changing room after a squash game you could always identify the surgeons because they were the ones with unsightly varicose veins. Knowing the risks of the operation to strip such veins they would never have the operation themselves but would happily advise their patients to do so. Sadly, after a couple of years David ceased communicating with AVMA and despite numerous attempts on my part to contact him I never heard from him again. At AVMA we speculated that perhaps he had been got at by the medical establishment or been sued for compensation himself? No doubt there was a much more innocent explanation.

Despite the help we were getting from a few friendly doctors the lack of medical expertise at AVMA continued to be a drawback. The number of cases with which we were dealing continued to increase and I still had a backlog from the 500 or so cases that had landed on my desk immediately after the launch. It was simply not possible for me to deal with the medical aspects of all the cases given that I had to undertake a substantial amount of reading for each one, and I could not telephone one of our small band of friendly doctors every time I did not understand something. And of course not having a medical background I often could not get to the bottom of the matter. At the same time, unless a case was clearly hopeless I had in most instances no option but to refer it to one of our equally small band of solicitors. That was obviously not satisfactory, firstly because it meant that I was referring far too many cases to solicitors than was necessary and furthermore the problem was simply passed to those solicitors who had no more medical expertise than I had.

The breakthrough, and probably the biggest breakthrough in AVMA's history, came when we received a grant from the Kings Fund. Apart from giving us the money to employ another worker, this had enormous significance. Remember that the Kings Fund, notwithstanding that we had been entertained with lovely cucumber sandwiches, had refused to fund us to set up the organisation. There were two reasons why this was such a major breakthrough. Firstly, the fact that the Kings Fund, a research foundation highly respected among healthcare professionals, was now prepared to back us, gave us a legitimacy and a profile which we had lacked up to then. The King's Fund was in effect saying that working for patient safety and at the same time helping victims of medical accidents, even if that sometimes meant helping them to sue doctors, was a good thing.

Secondly it enabled us to recruit Julia Cahill. As I have indicated, what we desperately needed at that time was medical expertise. I had enjoyed becoming familiar with medical terms as well as learning about various medical problems. Indeed I believe that I was beginning to kid myself that I was a medical expert. (I did not, I am pleased to say, go as far as one of our solicitors who, when he became highly experienced in medical negligence, included on his letter head the word "neurosolicitors"!) My family did, however, begin to say that the only reason that I had become involved with AVMA was to get even with my older brother the Obstetrician.

Having no in-house medical experience at AVMA was a dangerous situation, and the sooner we recruited a medic of some sort the better. Our Trustees and I had agreed that we should recruit a Deputy Director. (At that time my title was Director. That title went through a number of changes. When AVMA became a company limited by guarantee in 1988 we realised that as Director there would be confusion with the Directors on the Board. Accordingly we changed my title to Executive Director. Later we were advised that even retaining the word Director in my title could make me liable as a Director in certain circumstances. In any event AVMA had grown and it was thought that we warranted the grander-sounding Chief Executive and that is what I became.)

What we wanted to recruit therefore was a Deputy Director who could be a support for me but one who had a medical background and could deal with the cases or at least give me advice when I was doing cases. If they had any legal training that would be a bonus. Even though we were not offering much of a salary – after all I was only on £11,000 a year – we had a large number of applicants. Two of the Trustees and I had arranged to do the shortlisting on a Saturday morning at the office in Stockwell. Only a few of the applicants had anywhere near the qualifications and experience we were looking for and we had quite a gruelling time going through them all and achieving a shortlist of five. With relief we came to the end. We were just packing up when we heard the door downstairs open and the rush of footsteps up the stairs. We looked at each other quite anxiously given the situation of the office and I was already kicking myself for not having locked the door.

A young woman came into the office, thrust an application into Peter Ransley's hand and fled. We were undecided as to what to do. The time for submitting an application had expired the day before. We had completed the shortlisting and were pretty tired. I think it was Peter who said that as we had the application we should at least look at it. It was from Julia Cahill. A simple glance at it showed that on paper at least she was exactly what we were looking for. She was a solicitor who had qualified in New Zealand. She had also before that been a practising physiotherapist. Quite clearly we had to interview her. Interviews took place the following week and it was soon obvious that there was no contest. Not only did Julia have the qualifications but she had the interest and commitment as well as an element of feistiness which would stand her in good stead with the battles which lay ahead for AVMA. She demonstrated this feistiness for the first time when she agreed to take the job only on condition that she was paid at the top of the salary range we were offering which was not what we had in mind!

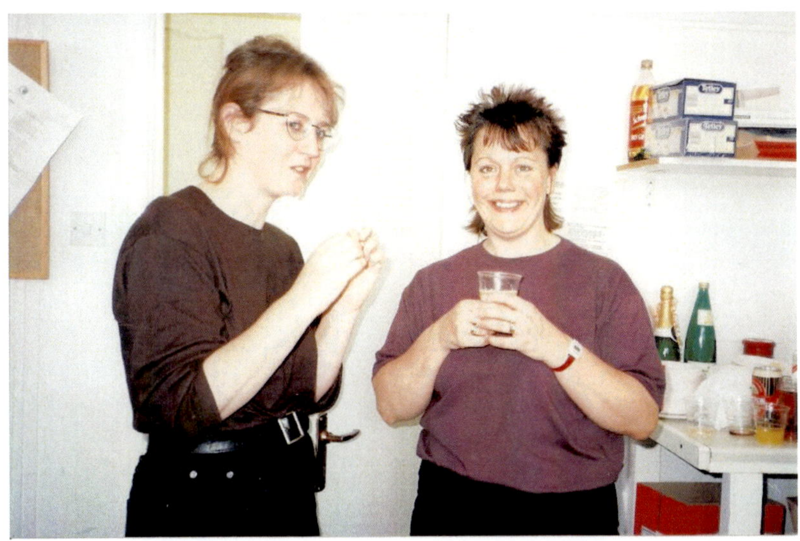

**Julia Cahill, left, AVMA's first Deputy Director**

Julia had a great and immediate effect on AVMA. The quality of our casework improved so that instead of having to pass almost every case to a solicitor Julia could do a preliminary medical analysis. I had of course been doing this, with the help of friendly doctors, but now this analysis was based on medical knowledge and could be done much more quickly. Passing cases straight on to solicitors had not in fact been a great advantage. To a large extent they could not do much more of an investigation than we could. What we, and they, needed was a full medical investigation by a doctor who was expert in the particular medical condition involved. But obtaining an expert's opinion cost money. Most clients were not in a position to pay. Legal Aid should have funded the obtaining of an expert's report. But that is where there was a Catch 22.

As I have explained in chapter 3 it was hardly ever possible to obtain a Legal Aid certificate without a medical expert's opinion. But to get such an opinion unless you had money you needed a Legal Aid certificate. The answer was, as I have indicated, to grant a Legal Aid certificate limited to obtaining an expert's report. But at that time the rules did not provide for such a thing as a limited Legal Aid certificate.

# Chapter 5
# Tackling the litigation problems

It was clear to us at that stage that the pressure for change would only come through improving the success rate of legal proceedings and the problem of improving legal aid support was AVMA's first big battle in the legal arena. It was essential that Legal Aid should be granted to investigate a potential claim. How did we approach it? AVMA co-ordinated a group of solicitors in our fledgling Lawyers' Support Group (see below) to approach the Law Society on the issue. After strong representations and much discussion the Law Society conceded. Certificates limited to obtaining an expert's opinion would be granted.

From that time the success rate of cases began to improve. The virtuous circle continued to expand. As solicitors gained more experience so their confidence and ability in the field grew. As that grew their success rate grew. And as their success rate grew they were willing to take on more cases. Furthermore, successful cases and AVMA itself were gaining publicity. As a result more people were either consulting AVMA or going direct to solicitors. Certainly the solicitors to whom we were referring cases were gradually becoming as expert as the solicitors acting for the defence organisations or hospitals.

There was, however, a downside. As the field of medical negligence became more popular more solicitors were jumping on the bandwagon by taking on medical negligence cases without the necessary experience or contact with AVMA. We began to see more clients who had been to a solicitor who had spent months if not years dealing with their case and who had eventually told them they did not have a case. If a client was then lucky enough to approach AVMA when we looked at what had been done by the solicitor it was clear that they did not have the faintest idea how to handle a complicated medical negligence case. They had wasted the time of a vulnerable client as well as much taxpayers' money.

AVMA tackled this in two ways. Firstly we began to run training courses for lawyers. At those courses we not only endeavoured to impart to solicitors the essentials of handling a successful medical negligence case but we also made it clear that unless solicitors were prepared to specialise and devote a substantial amount of their caseload to medical negligence they should not undertake the work at all. As far as we were concerned dabbling in medical negligence could do more harm to victims than not taking on their case at all. Our views on these matters led to some interesting debates and sometimes challenging situations. One of the first lectures on medical negligence which I gave was at a seminar run by the Legal Action Group. By that time there was already considerable interest in this new branch of the law and a number of solicitors attended hoping to learn how to run these cases or to run them better, which was always the aim of LAG seminars in relation to all aspects of litigation. This one took place in the North of England at Old Trafford Cricket ground. One of the points I made very strongly in my lecture was that it was no good for a solicitor to dabble in medical negligence and AVMA would certainly not refer a client to a dabbler. We believed that in order to acquire and maintain the expertise necessary to run a case properly, and to be any match for the expertise of the defence solicitors, a plaintiff solicitor would have to devote at least 40% of his or her caseload to medical negligence.

At the close of the seminar a local solicitor approached me. He was quite complimentary about my lecture but said that it was the first time he had paid good money to attend a course and been told by the lecturer that he should cease doing the kind of work he had come to learn about.

Slowly we began to build up what we called our Lawyers' Service. This comprised two elements, the Lawyers' Support Group and our Solicitor's Referral Panel. We considered that it was vital that there was a clear differentiation between these two sections and chose the names of the sections carefully. The Support Group was meant to indicate that members were supporting us in our endeavours to secure justice for victims of medical accidents and AVMA was in return supporting them. They were supporting AVMA because, not being involved in the day-to-day conduct of cases, we needed their feedback and help as much as they needed us. Later they were also supporting us financially through their membership fee. We on the other hand were supporting lawyers by helping them to handle cases for victims of medical accidents generally and our clients in particular. Members of the Support Group were also expected to help their colleagues who also were members. I believe that AVMA broke new ground in the way lawyers operated. Certainly at that time the vast majority of solicitors in most if not all fields kept their expertise and their knowledge to themselves, regarding them as trade secrets. Because the lawyers who joined us were absolutely committed to the idea of helping victims of medical accidents, they were prepared to help each other in achieving that aim. It was certainly the first time in my experience that lawyers who were considered to be experts in their field were prepared to exchange their trade secrets. This exchange took place not only with their expert colleagues but also with any lawyer who was a member of our service, even if far less experienced. I believe that this happened not only because of the lawyers' commitment but because of the excitement and often delight that was generated by being involved in what was fast becoming a brand new legal specialty.

The Solicitors' Referral Panel was something entirely different. It simply comprised those solicitors whom we regarded as competent to deal with our clients' medical negligence cases. Being a member of the Support Group did not automatically qualify solicitors in that way and we made no charge for being on our referral panel.

Many of the lawyers who were the first members of the AVMA Lawyers' Service made their names in medical negligence litigation through their involvement in medical negligence and membership of AVMA. I have already mentioned Anne Winyard who went on to become a partner in Leigh Day & Co, one of the leading medical negligence firms in England. As I have mentioned, David Body was working for a city firm, Halls, when he made contact with me. Again his obvious commitment persuaded me that he would provide the service victims needed, notwithstanding that at that stage he had no experience even in personal injury litigation let alone medical negligence. He subsequently became a partner in Irwin Mitchell, also one of the leading medical negligence firms, and has been involved in many of the seminal medical negligence cases over the years.

When we first established the Support Group we made no charge as we did not feel entitled to do so. By 1983, having developed some expertise we felt we were able to levy a small charge. Our first charge was £25 a year. While we were able to provide the lawyers with some benefit we did not feel that such benefit warranted a substantial fee. After all, we were all learning together. When, for example, we furnished a solicitor with the name of an expert in those early days it was like as not to be someone whom another member of the service had referred to us. Nor were we in a position to give any kind of endorsement of the expert. So it was very much a two-way process and the charge we made was as much a donation to the work of the charity as a charge for services rendered. By the end of 1983 we had 64 paid-up members.

We also had to be very careful to make it quite clear that membership of the Lawyers' Service was not an entitlement to be on our solicitors' panel and have cases referred to the them by AVMA. The last thing we wanted was for solicitors to think that their subscription entitled them to receive referrals. Throughout my time at AVMA this was a very tricky situation. It was particularly so when the service had developed so that we felt able to charge a commercial rate. Many solicitors, however much we stressed to the contrary, continued to believe that membership of the service was a gateway to receiving cases.

The referring of cases was dealt with entirely separately. Initially, I simply referred cases to solicitors I personally knew and felt I could trust. As our expertise developed we were able to assess whether a solicitor would be able to handle a medical negligence case properly. We therefore formally set up the Referral Panel. In those early days there were no problems. It was acknowledged that AVMA knew more about medical negligence than solicitors, especially since we had the medical expertise of Julia Cahill. Whilst our criteria for membership of the panel were not formally spelled out, what we were looking for were at least three things: First and foremost that a solicitor recognised that dealing with a medical negligence case actually required a particular expertise which was different from that required in dealing with a personal injury case; secondly that the solicitor was prepared to get to grips with the medical issues – that meant no longer relying slavishly on the medical expert but being prepared to read up on the medical issues involved, to instruct an expert in detail as to those issues and to be prepared to analyse the report received and challenge the experts where necessary; finally, we needed solicitors who would have empathy with the client. From our experience by the time we set up the panel, with patients who had suffered a medical accident, or their relatives where the accident had resulted in death, we were aware that anyone who had been through the mill of a medical accident was in a particularly vulnerable situation. Apart from the usual trauma suffered by an accident victim, they believed that they had been badly let down by the professional they most trusted. It was essential that the new professional they were asked to deal with would be able to give them confidence that they would not be let down again. In this connection one of the things that AVMA was insistent on was that it was as bad to encourage a victim to pursue a case without foundation as it was to fail to pursue a case which had promise.

It was, however, the issue as to whether there was a difference between medical negligence and "ordinary" personal injury litigation that led to the greatest difficulties for those solicitors who considered themselves experts in the latter. With hindsight it was certainly a mistake to refer to "ordinary" personal injury. We at AVMA always put the word in quotation marks and our aim was simply to underline the difference between what were clearly two different branches of the law albeit with many similarities. Nevertheless, expert personal injury lawyers could hardly have been expected to take kindly to such an epithet given that non-medical negligence personal injury cases could on occasion be every bit as challenging as medical negligence cases.

An opportunity to bring this issue into the open arose with the formation of the Association of Personal Injury Lawyers (APIL) in April 1990. Experienced personal injury (PI) lawyers had long been concerned about the harm that was done to their reputation by the fact that most solicitors thought they could do personal injury work and many of them did it extremely badly. Many members of the public were consequently ill-served, with cases taking years to complete, many being lost when they should have been won and thousands of cases being settled for substantially less than they were worth. The reputation of personal injury lawyers generally suffered accordingly.

Partly inspired by the example of AVMA a number of senior personal injury lawyers led by Michael Napier of Irwin Mitchell, a leading firm if not the leading firm in PI work, and John Melville-Williams QC, proposed setting up an organisation to address the problem. I was invited to stand for the Executive. Before agreeing to do so I had to clarify for the AVMA Trustees whether there was a conflict of interest. Mike Napier assured me that the new organisation would be very careful not to tread on AVMA's toes and to this end would exclude clinical negligence from its remit. The Trustees were therefore quite encouraging and I put my name forward and was duly elected to the Executive. I was re-assured when the key objectives of the organisation were agreed. They were:

- The promotion of full and just compensation for all types of personal injury.
- To promote wider redress for personal injury in the legal system.
- The development and promotion of expertise in the practice of personal injury law.
- Campaigning for improvements in personal injury law.
- The promotion of health and safety to alert the public to hazards.
- To provide a communication network to our members.

It will be seen that the focus of AVMA was the victims and their needs whereas APIL's approach, while also victim-based, was more on law, compensation and the expertise of lawyers. From the outset, however, there were members of the Executive who argued strongly against excluding medical negligence. While the majority of the Executive were those who were not only well-disposed towards AVMA but also recognised that damaging AVMA was not in the interests of victims, it was not difficult for me to hold the line. Gradually, however, APIL grew and became more powerful and new Executive members managed to have the exclusion removed. Today APIL includes medical negligence in all its activities including running courses in clinical negligence in direct competition with AVMA.

Meanwhile AVMA's Support Group and the Referral Panel forged ahead. The number of firms who were prepared to pay a

commercial sum to join the Lawyers' Service increased
exponentially as it became clear that with the right expertise
medical negligence cases could succeed. It seemed that we had hit
on something that would help victims in two ways. Firstly, and
most importantly, more lawyers would have the expertise to
support them and win their cases. Secondly, the service was a
source of funding for AVMA which would enable us to provide
victims with a better service.

Emboldened by this, and again with both objectives in mind,
we decided, in 1989, to hold a medical negligence conference for
lawyers. This was an enormous gamble. Although our reputation
was growing we were by no means sure that lawyers would be
prepared to pay good money to attend a conference organised by
people who had no track record in organising conferences. Not
only did we not have a track record, we had no experience. We
therefore believed that the only way to give credibility to the
conference and so encourage attendance was to have a least one
high-profile speaker, respected by lawyers. One of our panel
solicitors, David Body, felt he had sufficient connection with Lord
Griffiths, a member of the Judicial Committee of the House of
Lords, to ask him if he would be the keynote speaker. Much to
our delight Lord Griffiths agreed. That did not guarantee a
successful conference but it certainly meant it was a viable
proposition.

Getting the other speakers was not too difficult as we knew
sufficient doctors and lawyers of calibre who would be prepared
to speak and would be an attraction. Indeed, doctors speaking at a
lawyers' conference would be a novel event in itself and we
concentrated on medical speakers. The conference, which was
held in Harrogate in March 1989, was a stunning success. Over a
hundred delegates attended and we made what was for us a great
deal of money. Furthermore, the buzz of excitement throughout
the conference was testament to how much the delegates enjoyed
it. This has been a feature of AVMA conferences ever since. One
very gratifying feature from our point of view was that the speaker
from the United States, a successful lawyer with a great deal of
experience in medical malpractice, as it is called there, strongly
endorsed our view that getting to grips with the medical issues
was fundamental to running a successful medical negligence case.
"It is unthinkable," he said during the course of his lecture, "for

lawyers not to have a solid medical grounding if they are to take on the medical profession."

The medical profession was not so welcoming. An article in *General Practitioner*, a free paper for the profession, the week after the conference, began "Any doctor attending last weekend's Action for Victims of Medical Accidents (AVMA) conference in Harrogate would be forgiven for having grave doubts about entering medicine." On the other hand, the conference enhanced AVMA's standing among the legal profession greatly. So much so that, soon after, the Law Society agreed to give us a small grant to encourage us to continue training solicitors in medical negligence litigation.

After that first conference the AVMA Conference became an annual event. Each year it attracted a larger audience and within a few years it had reached a stature whereby it was considered by any lawyer serious about undertaking medical negligence work that attendance at the AVMA conference was essential. The fascinating aspect of the conferences for me was the attitude of those who attended. Of course they were paying a substantial amount to attend (although AVMA always kept the attendance fees well below those charged by commercial organisations) and they expected, if not demanded, the highest standard of lecturers who would provide them with the wherewithal to conduct their cases better and hopefully maximise their profits. Nevertheless the spirit of those attending was essentially one of wishing to help those who had suffered medical accidents and to enhance patient safety by preventing and reducing the number of accidents. Given that that would mean less work for them some might find it surprising but it supported my view of the public-spirited nature of most of those who practised in that discipline.

I gained this impression not only from the conversations I both had and overheard throughout the two days of the conferences. It was also from the way in which lectures not on the law or conduct of cases were received. Our conferences, unlike other law conferences, always included topics which went to the greater understanding of the social and ethical issues surrounding the problem of medical accidents as well as client care and these were always well received and certainly not seen as a waste of time. So, for example, we had representatives of Community

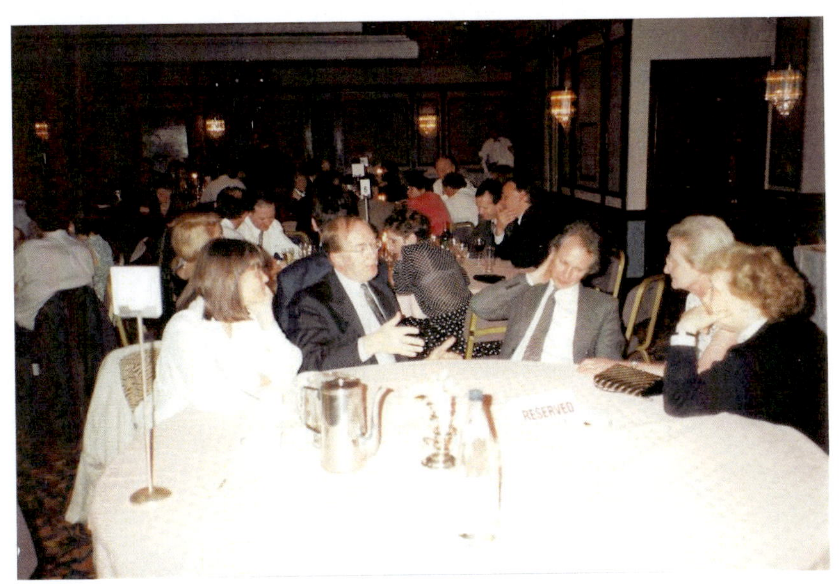

AVMA Conference, Brighton 1994.
Three Trustees from R to L –
Jean Robinson, Barbara Banks and Charles Vincent

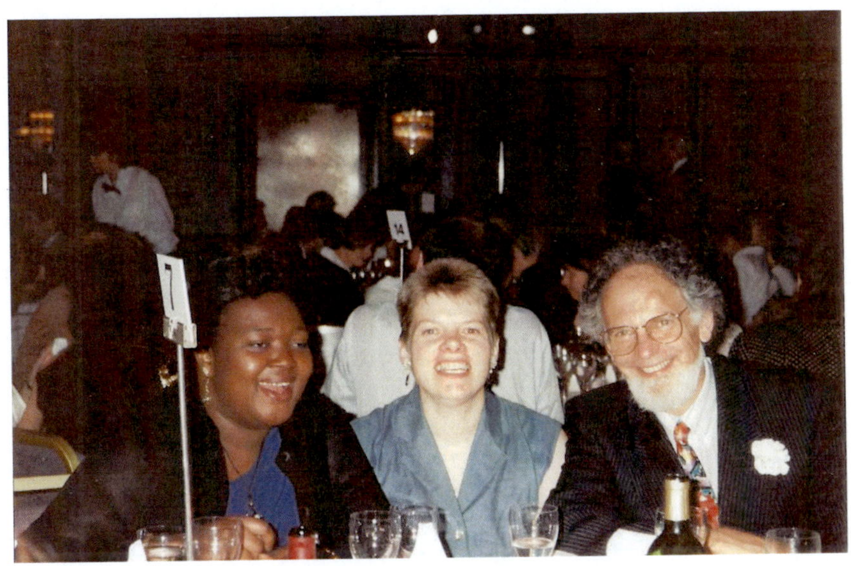

The author with two AVMA workers,
Pat Osinayke (L) and Georgina Tansley
at the Brighton Conference 1994

organisations to speak about how they approached the issue and Hospital Managers to speak on their perspectives as well as in later years lectures specifically on patient safety.

We always tried, at these conferences, to have an after dinner speaker who would both be an attraction because he or she had something important to contribute as well as being entertaining. Two such speakers at opposite ends of the spectrum will always be an abiding memory for me. At one early conference I invited a visiting American malpractice attorney, of considerable renown in his country, to give the after dinner speech. I carefully explained to him that the audience would want to learn about the American malpractice experience from a practical point of view but as it was an after-dinner speech we would want it to be light-hearted and entertaining as well as informative and, hopefully, instructive. In the event he decided to present an erudite and very heavy treatise which lasted rather a long time. This resulted in some extremely bad behaviour on the part of some of the delegates. At the back of the room was a group of young male lawyers who had obviously imbibed too much alcohol during the dinner and were relaxing after a heavy conference day. As the speaker droned on they began to heckle, and, egged on by each other they began to make comments in louder and louder voices. I had much sympathy with their impatience but none with their behaviour which everyone else found quite disgusting. The speaker left the dinner immediately after his presentation and although I wrote apologising for the rudeness of the small group I never heard from him again. Hopefully those young men are today experienced and useful medical negligence lawyers who look back on that incident with shame.

What a contrast to George Bonney who also did the honours in one of the early conferences. He was an Orthopaedic Surgeon, highly respected by his colleagues, who had done wonderful work for victims of medical negligence for some years. He had a lovely personality and much humanity and we thought he would be an excellent choice as an after-dinner speaker. So it turned out, although not after some heart-stopping moments for me. I sat next to him throughout the dinner and observed with mounting concern the amount of alcohol he managed to consume. It was true the quality of his conversation did not falter but he was then quite elderly and I was worried lest he would not be able to stand never mind deliver an entertaining speech. The time came for his speech and after I introduced him in glowing terms he stood up. To me he appeared a little unsteady but I am not sure anyone else noticed, although the fact that I took his arm as he stood probably was not missed. He looked around the room. For fully a minute, although it seemed like an hour to me, he said nothing and my heart sank.

I need not have worried. He then launched into a most brilliant speech which combined the wisdom of a great and humane doctor with the wittiness and timing of a stand-up comedian. During the speech he made a swingeing attack on the Thatcher government which he considered was harming the practice of medicine which went down extremely well with the audience. It was certainly the best after-dinner speech AVMA had produced and I doubt whether it will ever be equalled.

Contributions like that only served to emphasise the quality of our conferences and as a result of their popularity they were able to have a major impact on improving not only the chances of securing justice for victims of medical accidents but of patient safety. Indeed as recently as 2008 a gynaecologist was quoted in the Guardian as saying that the threat of "malpractice" suits made her a better doctor. (*The Guardian* G2 4th October 2008)

On the other side of our work with lawyers, the Referral Panel began to make a major impact. All solicitor members of the Lawyers Service of course wanted to be on the panel so that they could increase their caseload of medical negligence cases. We were, however, determined to maintain the highest possible standards. After all, we were at heart a patient's body, working for patient safety. There was little point in putting our clients in touch with a solicitor who was not going to do the very best for them. While at one point there were nearly a thousand firms who were members of the Lawyers' Service, the number of referral solicitors was always considerably fewer.

This policy paid off in another respect. In 1999 the Legal Services Commission had replaced the Legal Aid Board, which had itself taken over conduct of Legal Aid from the Law Society. In order to ensure that public money was only paid to competent medical negligence solicitors the Commission made it a requirement that only approved solicitors would be allowed to conduct legal aid cases. It agreed, however, that solicitors on

AVMA's panel would be automatically approved. This was another demonstration of the standing AVMA had by then reached in the legal world.

Another way which we found to increase the expertise of lawyers handling medical negligence cases and at the same time increase our income was the production of a journal. What a cheek! A small charity with no publication and little journalistic experience and a tiny staff already heavily committed, would set out to publish a journal which would come out regularly and would attract sufficient subscribers not only to support the journal but actually to make a profit. I suspect that if we had had more experience we would never have risked it. But by 1990 when we were contemplating this step we already had a large and loyal following in the Lawyers' Service and I must admit that we were relying on the adage coined by Keith Miles our Lawyers Service manager and later Deputy Director that our members would "come to the opening of an envelope"! We were satisfied that medical negligence had become a legal discipline in its own right and as such needed its own journal.

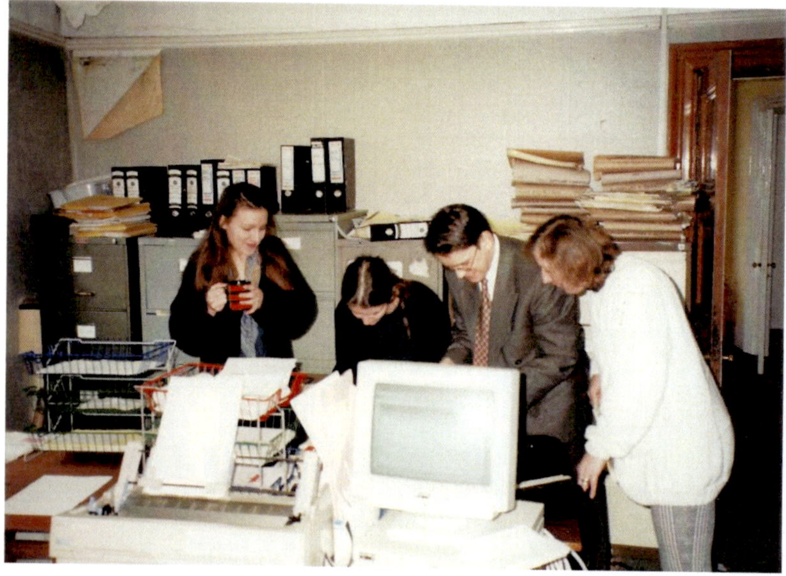

**The Lawyers' Service at work in AVMA's Forest Hill office –
From L-R, Paula Sparks, Tracy Minns, Keith Miles, Deputy
Director, Pauline Phillips**

So in 1990 we launched the *AVMA Medical and Legal Journal*. From the start it aimed to contain articles of the highest calibre, equally split between medical and legal. What the lawyers found particularly valuable were the cases we reported. We were at last able to achieve an important aim set out in our first press release: **"Out-of-court settlements** – It would assist claimants to know previous settlements and these should be published." As nobody else would publish them we were doing so ourselves. Once again we were only able to achieve this through the co-operation of our lawyers. They sent in details of their cases, both those tried and those settled and we never had a shortage of these.

Once more we became victims of our own success. The journal had only been published for a few years when the Royal Society of Medicine decided that they wanted to publish a journal dealing with clinical risk which was a new buzzword in the NHS. I saw the danger immediately. Clinical risk of necessity covered both patient safety and medical negligence, the core of the AVMA journal. The Society, with its massive resources and its connection with the members of the medical profession would be able to produce a journal which would be far more attractive to the health carers, both clinicians and administrators, than our journal. Both our teaching resource and our funds would be seriously threatened. Fortunately the driving force behind the new journal was Roger Clements, who was now heavily involved as an expert in medical negligence cases. He had always been a good friend to and supporter of AVMA. I immediately contacted him and expressed my fears. I don't think he had realised the implications of what he was proposing and he assured me that he had no wish to harm AVMA nor indeed medical negligence lawyers. He agreed to think about it.

Not long afterwards he contacted me with a proposal for merging the two journals. I knew that it was unlikely that I would be able to stop the new project going ahead and even if I did so another prestigious body would soon see the possibilities. I decided to agree to the proposal and get the best terms I could. Of course the Royal Society had much to gain as they would have a ready-made distribution list which was not insignificant. The merger turned out to be extremely successful for AVMA. We acquired a new readership among health carers who became familiar with and better able to understand the aims of AVMA and the journal continued to be lucrative for us.

# Chapter 6
# Money worries

Successful conferences had another important consequence. I had long since realised that AVMA was not the kind of sexy charity that would attract massive donations from the public. After all, we were perceived as attacking the medical profession, and the NHS and the media had no hesitation in portraying us as depriving the Health Service of money which should have been spent on patients. It was not surprising therefore that when we were lucky enough to win a spot on BBC radio for a public appeal we received only £4,000 when the average for that kind of appeal was about £15,000, and £3,500 of that £4,000 came from a Trust which supported our aims.

As a result, throughout my time as Chief Executive shortage of funds was a serious problem. On at least one occasion the Trustees were considering serving redundancy notices on all the staff as we did not appear to have sufficient funds to continue. We also had to consider major changes in our methods of working in order to save money. I and the staff were implacably against the options which were suggested: Firstly it was to charge clients. We considered that that would fundamentally change the relationship between AVMA and victims, apart from denying help to those who would often be in most need of it. Secondly it was to refer anybody who contacted us directly to competent solicitors. That would mean that we would be unable to assess the nature of the case or give the client assistance and advice outwith the legal possibilities and again would be contrary to our aims. And finally it was suggested that we simply close the phone lines from time to time so as not to take on any new clients. Sadly, we did have to adopt that option for short periods on occasion but this did not greatly relieve our financial pressures. These dilemmas were not resolved until some time after I left AVMA.

It was therefore clear to me that unless we generated our own funds we would never be able to grow into an organisation that could actually effect change. The only thing we had to sell was our services to Lawyers. Like our Lawyers Service our Annual Conference became a major source of income for the charity.

Our reliance on money from lawyers for a large part of our income – at one point as much as 70% of our funds came from that source in one way or another – was a matter of considerable concern for me and the Board of Trustees of AVMA for two reasons. Firstly, there was the danger that Government, the health carers and the public would see us simply as an extension of the legal profession. Given that one of our main aims was to influence health carers in order to change their attitudes and their culture, and that we needed the public to understand that we were an entirely independent organisation fighting for the rights of patients and public as well as patient safety, that would not be helpful. The second cause for concern was that we knew that a number of factors were bound to result in the reduction of our income from lawyers. The very fact that we were determined that only experts would do the work would reduce the number of firms that would require our services. This was exacerbated when the Legal Aid Commission introduced very strict requirements for solicitors who wished to conduct medical negligence work under Legal Aid. In addition the Commission was making it more and more difficult to get legal aid and reducing the fees payable for much of the legal aid work. As a result, many firms were deciding that the game was not worth the candle. The third factor was that, having created the new specialty of medical negligence law, commercial organisations as well as APIL were increasingly getting in on the act and organising conferences in competition with AVMA's as well as providing experts and training in this area.

This dilemma over the origin of our funds was not confined to income from lawyers. Like many other charities we agonised over the ethics of accepting certain funds which might run contrary to our principles. Indeed this has been a major debate in the voluntary sector world and I recall many years ago going to a lecture organised by the National Council for Voluntary Organisations (NCVO) on the topic. For us the issue blew up over seeking support from drugs companies. At a heated debate at a Trustees' meeting a majority on the Board voted to approach these companies notwithstanding my advice to the contrary. Our finances at that stage were in a very precarious state and our Treasurer in particular was convinced that the only way we could remain solvent was to approach drugs companies as a matter of urgency. Of course we did not know whether they would in fact support us and the worst of all worlds would have been if they turned us down.

In the event the approach was not made – not at that time anyway. When I reported the decision to our staff there was consternation. They were unanimously of the view that not only would it be ethically unacceptable but there would be a major loss of confidence in AVMA in many members of the public particularly those who wished to seek our advice. The main plank of their argument was that many of our cases were caused or could be caused by the very drugs manufactured by the companies from whom we would be seeking support. It was clear that there would be at best great resentment among the staff and at worst some form of revolt which might lead to the loss of valuable employees. I took this view back to the next Trustees' meeting and after another debate, even more heated than before because some Trustees could not accept that the staff should decide policy, the decision was overturned. Sadly, as a result our Treasurer, a good friend and an important member of the Board, resigned.

I digress to tell the story of one way which I did find to inject some money, albeit hardly a fortune, into the charity. Desperate times require desperate measures. We are all guilty, from time to time, of making extravagant claims or statements which, if we had thought about them calmly, we might have thought better of uttering. Often they have a nasty habit of coming home to roost.

In this connection an abiding memory with me is the incident in the film *Cool Hand Luke* when Paul Newman, in prison for the first time and wanting to impress his jail-hardened fellow inmates, suddenly said "I can eat twelve dozen hard-boiled eggs in a sitting." Some time later, after the whole prison has laid their meagre savings in bets on his ability to do so, we see him lying on his back on a table, stomach horribly distended, sweat pouring from him trying to empty his weary mouth which is stuffed with egg number one hundred and twenty-five, while a friend waits to push in number one hundred and twenty-six.

This image came into my head again as I approached the twenty-fourth mile of the London Marathon.

In one of those expansive and optimistic moments, in September 1990, at the age of 51, I announced that I was going to run the Marathon to raise funds for AVMA. Little did I know what was really involved. I realised that I would have to do some training but having been a regular jogger for many years that seemed a fairly reasonable requirement. What turned out to be different about training to run twenty-six miles on a fixed date is the lack of choice. Once on what is literally a treadmill of training you cannot get off unless you decide to give up altogether.

That meant that throughout the winter, whatever the weather, I found myself donning my running gear and going out to do my stint – first five miles, later ten miles and, eventually, over fifteen miles at a time. This has to be done five or six times a week and you dare not take a break. Mind you, you do meet other fanatics when you go out in that kind or weather. I recall very early one Sunday morning when the snow was lying thick on the ground, and I was gingerly picking my way along the frozen surface, terrified lest I slip and break a leg (the fear, or course, being not about the pain or damage but the inability to continue my training). I caught up with another runner who seemed to be running even more awkwardly. We got chatting and I learned that he was a boxer. He had his weigh-in for a fight later that day and was obliged to lose four pounds. Not only did he have the usual layer of clothes on to protect against the cold and the biting wind that was blowing, but he also informed me that under his track suit he was wearing a dustbin liner to make him sweat!

By the time the race came round I felt only semi-prepared. For various reasons I had been unable to complete the full training schedule recommended by the race organizers. The farthest I had run in training was sixteen miles. What was I going to feel like when I entered the unknown? The start of the race was wonderful. All those thousands of people – different shapes, sizes and standards of fitness; all committed to one objective and with a terrific spirit. Once out on Greenwich Park, it was the spirit of the watching crowds which was so impressive. Nobody who has not run the Marathon can know what an uplifting feeling it is to have that happy, cheering, supportive mass of people willing you on.

Having friends on the route is a bonus. At seven miles, just when I was beginning to feel a little alone, I heard my name shouted and there was someone I actually knew – fantastic! I was expecting the main support from AVMA to be gathered at a pub (where else?) on Tower Bridge at the twelve-mile mark. That was my first objective. As I reached them I was feeling so fit that I flashed past them too fast for them even to aim their cameras! But I was filled with a glow of achievement. The halfway mark came and went in under two hours and I was beginning to feel that not only would I actually finish but I would do it in fine fettle.

The Marathon knows better! Almost on cue as I passed my limit of sixteen miles, I began to feel the strain. At that point I caught up with a woman quite a bit older than me and as I still had a little breath spare for talking I muttered something like "it's beginning to get slower, isn't it?". She cheered me up greatly by replying that, actually, she was getting faster!

The Isle of Dogs is usually the graveyard of the race and so it nearly proved for me. By eighteen miles, my legs were telling me quite clearly that they had had enough and they were not going to carry on with this crazy game anymore. I was very inclined to listen. Eight more miles to go – more than I usually run when I am feeling totally fit – impossible. Forget the sponsorship money, forget the pride – just have a rest.

Three things sustained me: One was the crowds. The spirit of the people – the original inhabitants of the Isle of Dogs that is, not the newly arrived Yuppies – was fantastic. They had prepared oranges and made some sandwiches to give to the runners, the children had sweets for us to suck which made a change from the water and sports drinks which were causing a strange sensation in the mouth. Cheering and cracking jokes they identified us by our running numbers and gave us individual support.

The second thing that kept me going was the knowledge that the AVMA staff were going to be at the twenty-two mile mark, having crossed from the other side of Tower Bridge. I couldn't let them down. Thirdly there was the sponsorship money. I had collected sponsors to the tune of £7000 and I could not run the risk of losing such a substantial sum. My legs seemed to be beating the refrain NE-VER A-GAIN, NE-VER A-GAIN. As I approached that point I could think of nothing else. Had my brain not been addled by exertion it would have been quite obvious to me that once the staff had been waiting in the pub at the twelve-mile mark for the one and a half hours it had taken for me to get round to that point they were not going to be inclined nor, indeed, in a state to make the journey across the bridge – and they weren't there when I arrived! Never, mind, they had served their purpose. I was at twenty-two miles and had only four miles to go. I was in real pain but, failing a complete breakdown, I knew I was going to finish.

Slower and slower, but the yards were being covered. I was into the Mall and my heart began to lift. My snail's pace began to quicken. Round to within sight of Big Ben and I was actually moving at a reasonable speed. My final determination was helped still further by yet another shout of my name and I was actually able to turn and wave to a friend.

Across the line. I had done it. AVMA was some thousands of pounds richer and I had an overwhelming sense of achievement and sharing in a great experience as well as gratitude to all those fantastic supporters.

# Chapter 7
# All change

The conversion of the vicious circle into a virtuous one had major consequences for the conduct of medical negligence litigation. One by one the old roadblocks began to be addressed.

*Legal Aid*

The Law Society's willingness to issue a Legal Aid certificate limited to obtaining the medical records and instructing a medical expert was a major breakthrough and the number of legal aid certificates issued rose exponentially. Between 1981 and 1999 (when the Legal Aid Commission decided once again to get tough about the issue of certificates) the number of certificates had increased from 800 to 12,000.

*Obtaining the medical records*

The difficulties with obtaining medical records prior to commencing action which had presented a Catch 22 situation were overcome as a result of the judgment in the case of *Hall v Wandsworth Health Authority* to which I have referred. In that case the court ordered not only that the records should be disclosed but that the defendants should pay the costs of the application. That meant that if hospitals or doctors failed unreasonably to disclose the records within a reasonable time they would invariably end up paying what could be quite substantial costs. This had a salutary effect on defendants.

This case also demonstrated how the tide was beginning to turn as far as the expertise of plaintiffs' solicitors was concerned. The solicitor acting for the plaintiff, Ann Winyard, felt sufficiently confident to argue the case herself against Robert Francis, a highly experienced QC, (subsequently a High Court Judge) regularly instructed by the Defence organisations. And she won. As a result of this decision it soon became the norm for medical records to be produced on request from a solicitor, though not always by return! The irony is that in the Wandsworth case, once the medical records were disclosed the plaintiff's solicitor was able to ascertain that there was in fact no basis for the claim and the patient did not proceed further with the case. You would have thought that the Defence organisations would have learned a lesson from that decision and the way in which it had led to the dropping of the claim. Sadly they did not. It took a long time before defence solicitors would almost always disclose the records on request.

*Exchange of medical reports*

But as important in ending trial by ambush was the Appeal Court decision in April 1987 in six cases involving four Health Authorities – Preston, Newham, Merton and Sutton and North West Surrey. These cases were consolidated under the title *Naylor and others v Preston Area Health Authority and others [1987] 2 AER 353*. The High Court held that both sides should exchange the reports of their medical experts. Until then, when plaintiff's solicitors *had* been able to obtain a satisfactory report they had been obliged to send it to the defendant's solicitors without being able to see any report the latter had obtained. I have previously explained the disadvantages for the plaintiff in not being able to see the defendant's medical report in advance of the trial. The court in *Naylor v Preston* held that it was unfair that the plaintiff should be disadvantaged by not seeing the defendant's medical report in advance of the trial and that there should be simultaneous exchange. The defendant's solicitors, and, as we shall see, the medical profession itself, saw this as so important that they appealed to the Court of Appeal. Unfortunately for them, and happily for the cause of victims of medical accidents, the court of Appeal endorsed the decision.

AVMA played an important part in this case. As I wrote in our Annual Report for 1986/88:

> "AVMA's role in that case was crucial. We co-ordinated the solicitors in six different cases involving the same procedural issue and ensured that the cases were presented in the best way. It was of course, AVMA which had created the conditions in which lawyers felt able to challenge a long-standing rule which had worked to the benefit of

those trying to deny justice to victims of medical accidents
by keeping the legal process as secretive as possible."

It is interesting to see the reference by the senior Appeal Court
Judge in that case, Sir John Donaldson, Master of The Rolls, to
the words of the Judge in an earlier medical negligence case.
Those words encapsulate the way in which this type of case used
to be conducted and why they came to be referred to as trial by
ambush: "In the result, the parties realised, soon after the case
began that they had misunderstood what the case was about. …It
was fought 'in the dark'. It lasted four weeks instead of the
allotted five days, which not only imposed great pressure of time
on all concerned but meant that the scheduling of the expert
witnesses was put quite out of joint. The Judge had nothing to
read beforehand except some pleadings which told him nothing.
The evidence of the Plaintiff's and Defendant's witnesses came
forward in no sort of order, sometimes by instalments. Nearly 150
pages of medical literature were put in without prior exchange or
any opportunity for proper scrutiny. All this could have been
avoided if there had been adequate clarification of the issues
before the Trial."

We have to ask why the medical profession saw this decision
as so damaging. After all, if the defendants wanted the truth to be
told then openness could do no harm. If the defendant's report
showed that there was negligence, then the defendants should
have been prepared to meet the claim. If on the other hand the
defendant's report showed no negligence and was well argued the
plaintiff's expert might well have conceded that that was the case.
If the experts remained in dispute it would be left to the court to
decide on the evidence given by the experts. One cannot help
being left with the impression that many in the medical profession
and their advisers were happy to rely on procedure to secure an
advantage. Indeed, notwithstanding all the progress that has taken
place in clinical negligence litigation since then, many claimant
solicitors are of the opinion that that is still the position.

We were delighted with a decision which went some way
towards creating a level playing field which would enable more
patients to achieve justice and we said so publicly. This led to an
astonishing leader in *Hospital Doctor* on the 23rd April 1987. Under
the heading "Justifying its own position" it referred to AVMA as

"malevolently anti-medical profession" and accused us, and me in particular, of encouraging a hostile atmosphere and being ourselves to blame for the reluctance of many doctors to be open with patients where a mishap has occurred. We could not let that go and I instructed solicitors to threaten libel proceedings by both AVMA and me personally. Negotiations eventually led to the publication of a fulsome apology in which the paper accepted, among other things, that AVMA was acting in the public interest.

This case also demonstrated how the AVMA lawyers were co-operating in the interests of victims generally because each of the cases was dealt with by a different solicitor but they co-ordinated their appeals and their arguments.

*Experts*

The Lawyers' Service was also one of the instruments whereby the pool of senior doctors prepared to give evidence on behalf of plaintiffs was increased. In addition it helped to educate doctors as to what was expected of them in that role. The members searched out doctors whom they thought, from their contacts, would be objective and persuaded them to act. After such doctors agreed and provided helpful reports the solicitors passed their names to AVMA to be included in the pool. The word also got around that there was good money to be made by acting as an expert witness and for some doctors that was an important attraction.

AVMA also had a major role to play in this connection. I spent a considerable amount of time writing to doctors and speaking at their events. The thrust of my argument was that doctors owed a duty to help patients who had been harmed while under medical care. It was often a member of the profession who had harmed them, and helping the patient to obtain compensation, which would make life easier for them, was also a part of care. After all, nobody else but a doctor could help them in that situation. One of my greatest triumphs in this regard was my talk at a conference of the Association of Surgeons in Training in September 1985. After the conference, which was the very first of that new association, the doctor who had organised it and had invited me to speak wrote about it, and the lessons he had learned, in *Hospital Doctor*. I quote: "A conference needs a threatening speaker. We thought we had one such in our legal debate in the Director of the Action for Victims of Medical Accidents. But after his carefully put plea on the rights of the patient the company turned, not on him, but on the representative of the MDU who found himself in the dock accused of encouraging the 'wall of silence' and the unnecessary delays."

The British Medical Association (BMA) also helped. They urged doctors to give reports for claimants on the somewhat questionable basis that they were in the best position to identify cases where negligence had not occurred and they could therefore prevent unjustified cases going ahead.

As a result of these initiatives, the attitudes of doctors began to change. AVMA and plaintiff solicitors did not only find it easier and easier to recruit medical experts; AVMA actually began to receive approaches from doctors themselves asking to be put on our panel. I personally found it quite amusing to see how difficult our Lawyers Service made it for doctors to get onto that panel. What a turn-up for the books! But we were determined to ensure that only experts who were well qualified to do the work and would give fair, unbiased reports supported by cogent evidence and argument were accepted. If doctors approached the task with the view that this was something that had to be done and that they would be entirely objective that could work against the victim. That is because doctors come with an inbuilt bias, and their objectivity would only be relative. What we were looking for were doctors who would approach the task from the victim's point of view. In other words they would be prepared to look for negligence whilst being entirely objective. That is what I labelled "partisan objectivity". We asked to see examples of applicants' reports as well as requiring references from solicitors. It was a measure of how things had changed that virtually all such applicants were prepared to comply with our requirements.

One development which was a consequence of this change was not entirely welcome. Because giving evidence in medical negligence cases had become popular and extremely well paid many doctors were anxious to put their information about in as many fora as possible. Both the Academy of Experts, a professional body established in 1977, and the Expert Witness Institute, a non profit-making body established in 1996, provided the names of experts in all types of litigation. They now began to attract medical experts in greater numbers.

AVMA had never objected to or been afraid of rivals. Our only concern was that those whom we were committed to helping, the victims of medical accidents themselves, should always benefit from any development. So, for example, when an organisation calling itself Action for Victims of Medical Blunders, aimed at helping victims, was set up our objection was not to the fact of their existence but whether, if victims approached them, they would get the help they deserved. This organisation was the brainchild of one of AVMA's disillusioned clients whom we advised did not have a case. He could not accept that and decided to set up in opposition (using a name not dissimilar to AVMA). Our concern was that without any expertise or understanding of the issues he did not have the ability to give those who needed help a comprehensive service which often might involve advising them not to litigate. This organisation simply referred enquirers direct to solicitors, most of whom were solicitors on our panel. In order to ensure that victims received the help they really needed we decided that any of our panel solicitors who accepted referrals from this organisation would be removed from our panel. A somewhat draconian remedy but one which we believed was essential in the interests of victims. All our panel solicitors understood our motives and, albeit in some cases somewhat reluctantly because it was another source of income, accepted the position. Whether because of this, Action for Victims of Medical Blunders soon disappeared.

Likewise when the Law Society and APIL set up their medical negligence panels we were concerned as to whether the requirements for being on those panels were sufficiently rigorous and aware of the needs of victims as to ensure that victims received the best advice available. Our concern in particular with these was that whilst AVMA's constituency was solely the individuals who might have been damaged whilst under medical care APIL's and the Law Society's primary constituency was the lawyers.

We had similar concerns with the providers of expert witnesses. Both the Institute and the Academy dealt with experts in all disciplines and did not concentrate, as AVMA did, solely on medical negligence. Whilst they had far greater financial resources than AVMA they were not involved in the area of medical negligence as we were beyond providing experts and did not have direct contact with those who had suffered a medical accident. They were, and are, concerned to ensure that their experts were technically competent in their fields and well trained in giving expert evidence. These are major requirements of course and ones which AVMA also required. But AVMA's dimension was greater. We were concerned to ensure that victims were properly treated. We had direct personal contacts with lawyers who used our experts and we required feedback from them about how experts actually performed both in writing reports and in the witness box. We also had direct contact with the experts in the particular cases and could discuss their reports with them and make clear what we were looking for.

This touches on the major issue of who is an expert which has yet to be resolved. The story goes that there was one particular expert who seemed to spend his life in the High Court. One of the judges soon noticed that whatever the kind of case he was trying, whether a road traffic accident, a divorce or a commercial dispute, this same expert appeared to give evidence. Eventually the Judge enquired of him, "Mr X, I see you're before me again. Can you explain in what particular area you are an expert?" My Lord," he replied, "I am an expert in giving expert evidence." This no doubt apocryphal story does illustrate the problem with which the judges have had to wrestle. The Courts and the Civil Procedure rules have gone to some pains to set out the role of an expert. The first guidance on this was set out by Cresswell J. in the *Ikarian Reefer [1993] 2 LILR 68*, at 81-82. Then there was a very clear re-statement of the principles in that guidance in the light of the Civil Procedure Rules by HH Judge Toulmin in *Anglo Group plc v Winther Brown & Co. Ltd. (2000)*:

> "In the case of The Ikarian Reefer [1993] 2 Lloyds Rep 68, at 81-82 Cresswell J analyzed the role of the expert witness.
>
> 1.    An expert witness should at all stages in the procedure, on the basis of the evidence as he understands it, provide independent assistance to the court and the parties by way of objective unbiased opinion in relation to matters within his expertise. This applies as much to the initial meetings of experts as to evidence at trial. An expert witness should never assume the role of an advocate.

2.   The expert's evidence should normally be confined to technical matters on which the court will be assisted by receiving an explanation, or to evidence of common professional practice. The expert witness should not give evidence or opinions as to what the expert himself would have done in similar circumstances or otherwise seek to usurp the role of the judge.

3.   He should co-operate with the expert of the other party or parties in attempting to narrow the technical issues in dispute at the earliest possible stage of the procedure and to eliminate or place in context any peripheral issues. He should co-operate with the other expert(s) in attending without prejudice meetings as necessary and in seeking to find areas of agreement and to define precisely arrears of disagreement to be set out in the joint statement of experts ordered by the court.

4.   The expert evidence presented to the court should be, and be seen to be, the independent product of the expert uninfluenced as to form or content by the exigencies of the litigation.

5.   An expert witness should state the facts or assumptions upon which his opinion is based. He should not omit to consider material facts which could detract from his concluded opinion.

6.   An expert witness should make it clear when a particular question or issue falls outside his expertise.

7.   Where an expert is of the opinion that his conclusions are based on inadequate factual information he should say so explicitly.

8.   An expert should be ready to reconsider his opinion, and if appropriate, to change his mind when he has received new information or has considered the opinion of the other expert. He should do so at the earliest opportunity.

9.   An expert witness should at all stages in the procedure, on the basis of the evidence as he understands it, provide independent assistance to the court and the parties by way of objective unbiased opinion in relation to matters within

his expertise. This applies as much to the initial meetings of experts as to evidence at trial. An expert witness should never assume the role of an advocate.

That analysis is extremely helpful but what it doesn't do is explain how an expert qualifies as such. As I have pointed out, it is possible to train experts in the art of giving expert evidence. But that does not make them an expert. And AVMA's fear was always that some artificial list of "experts" would be created, whether by the Courts, the Law Society, the Bar Council or indeed some specific body created for the purpose, which would be the final arbiter as to who would be entitled to give expert evidence in any type of case.

That list might not only include, insofar as medical negligence is concerned, people who had jumped through all the hoops but also those who felt that they owed their allegiance to their profession rather than to looking to do justice. It might also exclude those who were not willing or able to commit themselves to whatever was required to enable them to qualify according to the arbitrary standards set up but were nevertheless ideal expert witnesses in their particular field of medicine – hugely experienced and highly respected in their discipline with a balanced view as to what is required of an expert in a medical negligence case whether instructed by the claimant or defendant. In the absence of any better system, the way in which AVMA investigated potential experts seems to me to be the only acceptable method in the interests of those who may have been injured in a medical accident. It would identify the only experts in whom patients would have confidence when they gave a negative report.

We had no doubt that both the Institute and the Academy were doing excellent work. Our concern was that inexperienced lawyers, who were unable to judge the quality of an expert's work, might select an expert from the panel of one of these institutions and be badly served by him or her. We accepted, however, that as with a number of other areas where rival organisations had developed, this was simply a result of our own success in bringing medical accidents onto the agenda. In the long run, public and patients could only benefit from this.

The increasing expertise of lawyers not only led to improvements in procedure but, combined with the increasing co-operation of doctors, soon began to show in the enhanced success in cases. It also began to expose the lengths that so many healthcare professionals as a whole were prepared to go to cover up the truth.

*Ackers v Wigan Health Authority[1991] 2 Med LR91* was a fascinating case in point. Mrs Ackers underwent a Caesarean birth. When she awoke from the anaesthetic she was in a terrible state. She said that she had been awake throughout the operation. She had felt the knife slicing into her and the baby taken out. She had been in absolute agony but had been unable to move a muscle or scream. When she reported this to the staff they all pooh-poohed her story and said she must have been dreaming because she had been anaesthetised.

She consulted Ann Alexander, a local solicitor who had undertaken a few medical negligence cases. Mrs Ackers was so convincing in her recollection of what had happened that Ann decided to take on the case even though she knew that a number of similar cases had been unsuccessful simply because the patient had not been believed. She instructed an obstetrician to advise her. He reported that it was possible for this to happen if the muscle relaxant which had been injected was strong enough to make her immobile but the anaesthetic was not strong enough to put her to sleep. He explained that anaesthetists were reluctant to give too strong a dose of anaesthetic for fear of harming the baby in the womb. If Mrs Ackers' story were true, then that is what must have happened. On the strength of that report, and believing strongly in her client's story, Ann was able to obtain legal aid to pursue the case. The defendant Health Authority defended on the basis that it was not possible that Mrs Ackers had been awake.

Unfortunately for the defendant, the operation had taken place during a cricket test match and Mrs Ackers was able to recall the conversation in the operating theatre about the match, even to the extent of remembering the score. The Judge was convinced and found in her favour. Whilst that was a great triumph for both Mrs Ackers and her solicitor, it was the consequences of that case that were of equal if not greater importance, certainly to the general public and indeed to the medical profession.

Firstly, a number of women consulted Ann with similar stories. The defendants in most of these cases simply accepted liability and paid compensation. Secondly, and most importantly, procedures were developed by the medical profession to enable anaesthetists to ensure that the anaesthetic given was adequate without harming the baby.

Two lessons can be drawn from this case. Firstly, it shows just how far doctors and other health carers were prepared to go to cover up negligence. It is obvious that obstetricians knew the risk and in rejecting Mrs Ackers' story on the basis that that complication simply could not happen, all the medical personnel involved were complicit in covering up what had happened. Secondly, that AVMA's work combined with litigation could lead to greater patient safety.

This issue of cover-up, not only by doctors but by all sections of the Health Service, loomed large throughout my time at AVMA. The Defence Organisations maintained, and continue to maintain, that they always advised doctors to be open when things went wrong. Indeed they point to the written advice sent to all their members. Nevertheless the main problem all our clients invariably came up against was obtaining the true facts. And the case of *Hall vs Wandsworth* to which I referred earlier shows quite clearly that the Defence organisations and their solicitors were not prepared to be open even going as far as the Appeal Court to try to preserve their right to secrecy.

One of the cases that demonstrates how important it was that only experienced solicitors conducted medical negligence cases is that of *Blackburn v Newcastle Health Authority October 1987*

On the 28th September 1976 Keith Blackburn went to Newcastle General Hospital (NGI) with breathing difficulties, was given pain killers and sent home. However, he collapsed in the hospital and was taken home by ambulance. On the night of the 29th/30th September he became worse and was taken to NGI by ambulance suffering from pneumonia and pleurisy. On the 23rd Dec 1976 he was discharged, grossly disabled in thought, movement and speech and with a childlike personality.

Keith's father consulted solicitors who wrote to the hospital on the 20th January 1977. The trial judge described their letter as "a most ingenuous letter". It did not actually make a claim but asked for disclosure of Keith's records which was refused. The solicitors did not pursue the claim because of legal aid difficulties.

In 1979 Keith's father instructed a second solicitors' firm who issued a writ that was not served but was renewed in 1980. On the 12 January 1981 a third solicitors' firm served a statement of claim which revealed that at that stage they "had no idea what had caused the plaintiff's serious incapacity" (according to the Judge who eventually tried the case).

Keith's father was determined to find out what had happened to his son in the three months that he was in the Newcastle hospital. He eventually made contact with AVMA who in 1986 referred him to one of their panel solicitors, Michael Napier of Irwin Mitchell. When he informed the defendant's solicitors that he had been instructed they immediately tried to strike the case out for want of prosecution. They failed because Keith was a person under mental disability and therefore not caught by the Limitation Act.

Mike Napier obtained such records as existed. He instructed a professor who was a great expert in this particular branch of medicine and nursing and as a result of his report and three further reports he obtained he was able to get the case to trial in 18 months, some twelve years after Keith's father had started to look for answers. The essence of the reports that were obtained was that the medical and nursing staff were negligent because they failed to admit Keith early enough, they used unsatisfactory ventilation equipment in intensive care and they allowed a tracheostomy tube to become blocked. In giving judgment for the plaintiff the judge said, "I am driven to the conclusion that the cause of the brain damage was the failure to clear the tube out as it should have been cleared out." He was awarded over half a million pounds.

One of my most used quotations in lectures given at conferences was from a letter written by a consultant to a GP who had referred a patient to him. The letter was found in the medical records when they were eventually disclosed to the patient's solicitor in a case that was being strenuously defended. It read: "Thank you very much for letting me know that you have seen [patient]. As you may already know I get a succession of ghastly cock-ups from casualty here as [other consultant] persistently refuses to refer patients through to us. I am astonished that he has not been sued before now but there it is."

"There it is." The doctor writing the letter was a member of the Council of one of the Defence Organisations but did not think it appropriate to take any action to prevent these "ghastly cock-ups". And, as I said in my lecture, "The doctor who operated, the doctor who referred and the consultant who wrote the letter all knew there had been a 'cock-up'. The only person who did not know was the patient. What is more, up to that point, and even for a while afterwards, the case continued to be defended. Not only that but, as far as I am aware, no action was subsequently taken to refer the errant Consultant to the GMC."

Even more culpable, perhaps, was the doctor who when asked why the result of the treatment is such a disaster would refer to the problem as "one of those things" or would give some innocent or confusing explanation which was often accepted by the patient. For example a consultant explained to the relatives of a patient who had died under an anaesthetic that she was a victim of Mendelssohn's syndrome. It was only when we had obtained the opinion of an independent expert that we learned that Mendelssohn's syndrome simply referred to the fact that there had been inhalation of vomit which can be, and usually is, caused by negligent behaviour by the anaesthetist.

Sadly, although less prevalent, this behaviour continues. As recently as 2008 the media reported a case where a woman had died during an operation and the husband was told that she had died from a rare condition during childbirth. Only at the inquest some four years later did he discover that the cause of death was an injection negligently given by the midwife.

Whilst the case of Sidaway (*Sidaway v Bethlem Royal Hospital Governors [1985] AC 871*) did not result in success for the patient it did have far-reaching implications for the improvement of compensation claims. Because the judgment went against the patient it was not realised at the time just how significant the judgments of two of the Law Lords in that case were and how they would influence the future conduct of doctors to the benefit of patients.

The issue involved in that case was that of consent by patients to treatment. AVMA had become aware in the couple of years that we had been dealing with cases just how little information was being given to patients by doctors about the treatments or operations that they were to undergo. The principle was well established that a doctor could not treat a patient without his or her consent. However if the patient did not understand the implications of the treatment was she or he in a position to give their consent? We were repeatedly seeing cases where a patient had had an operation where the doctor had acted perfectly properly but the result was a disaster. If the patient had had no alternative but to undergo the operation then the fact that the result was unsuccessful, or worse still, left the patient in a poorer condition than before could not be a cause for complaint. But if the patient in fact had had a choice as to whether to undergo the operation that should have been an entirely different matter. So many times we would hear a patient say, "If I had known there was a possibility of this happening I would never have agreed to have the operation."

In the United States the judges had addressed this problem by developing the doctrine of "informed" consent. In other words a doctor was required to explain to a patient exactly what was involved in a treatment and what the complications might be. If the doctor did not do so and one of the known possible complications resulted, leaving the patient in a worse condition than before, the doctor would be just as liable for compensating the patient as they might have been had they actually botched the treatment. The British courts set their face against this doctrine. In the few cases that came before them based on this concept their attitude was always that if a patient had signed a form of consent, however little information had been given to them, the doctor could not be liable. Basically, they were adopting the hallowed principle that "doctor knows best".

AVMA began to campaign on the issue. As far as we were concerned this was a fundamental issue of patients' rights and patient safety. How could a person be said to have consented if they did not know what was involved? The medical profession, ably supported by their defence organisations, fought back. Whether I addressed the issue in public at conferences on medical negligence, or in private discussions with doctors or their representatives, the response was always the same. How could the amount of information the patient required be assessed? They scorned the American system where they claimed that patients were often accompanied by their lawyers when the doctor explained the implications of a proposed operation and the form of consent was drafted by lawyers and could consist of as much as fourteen pages.

Then came the case of Mrs Sidaway. Mrs Sidaway had suffered from recurring pain in her neck, shoulder and arm. She had undergone one operation which had given her relief for a while. When the pain began to increase again she returned to see the consultant neurosurgeon who had operated on her before. He advised her to have a repeat operation. What he did not tell her was that even if the operation were carried out with due care and skill there was a 2% chance of damage to the nerve root and spinal cord. In the event that was what happened and Mrs Sidaway was left severely disabled. She complained that she would never have had the operation had she known of the risk.

It was difficult for anyone to have disagreed with that assertion at least with hindsight. At the trial when asked what she would have done had she been told she replied that "I would 'ave put on me coat and gone 'ome." Nevertheless the Judge found in favour of the defendants. Mrs Sidaway appealed to the Court of Appeal. There too her claim was rejected. She was given leave to appeal to the House of Lords. I went to meet her after the Court of Appeal decision and pending the House of Lords hearing. I found her to be a delightful woman who was really distressed that she had not been warned of the possible consequences of the operation and emphatic that had she been she would not have undergone the operation had she known the risks. Although she had been suffering pain it was not enough to disable her. Indeed, she told me that just before she went into hospital for the operation she had been in the process of making a new dress for the Xmas Eve dance she was going to attend with her husband. Yes, she was in pain from time to time, but it didn't stop her dancing!

Sadly, all five of the Law Lords who heard the appeal were agreed that it should be rejected. (*Sidaway v. Bethlem Royal Hospital Governors [1985] AC 871*). As so often happens, however, the reasoning for the rejection was not the same on the part of every Law Lord. The appellant's argument was that the Bolam test (see chapter 3), which placed the decision as to what action to take wholly in the hands of a responsible doctor, should be confined to treatment and should not apply to giving advice or warnings. The latter were more a matter of practical common sense and the views of the patient. Three of the Law Lords rejected that argument out of hand. However, Lord Scarman and Lord Bridge, whilst finding that in this particular case the doctor had done what was necessary, nevertheless went a considerable way towards demolishing the Bolam test with regard to advice. Lord Scarman said as follows: "I am satisfied, for reasons which I shall develop, that the trial judge and the Court of Appeal erred in law in holding that in a case where the alleged negligence is a failure to warn the patient of a risk inherent in the treatment proposed, the 'Bolam test', to which I shall refer in detail at a later stage of my speech, is to be applied. In my view the question whether or not the omission to warn constitutes a breach of the doctor's duty of care towards his patient is to be determined not exclusively by reference to the current state of responsible and competent medical opinion and practice at the time, though both are, of course, relevant considerations, but by the court's view as to whether the doctor in advising his patient gave the consideration which the law requires him to give to the right of the patient to make up her own mind in the light of the relevant information whether or not she will accept the treatment which he proposes."

Lord Bridge did not go quite as far but he did say in relation to the Bolam test, "But I do not see that this approach involves the necessity to 'hand over to the medical profession the entire question of the scope of the duty of disclosure, including the question whether there has been a breach of that duty."

In an article in the *Journal of the Royal Society of Medicine* (Vol 79 December 1986) Lord Scarman made clear what he thought the position after Sidaway was. After making some preliminary observations about the standard of the duty of care with regard to "advice" as opposed to diagnosis and treatment, where the law was settled, he continued: "I ask myself in the light of the Sidaway decision whether the so-called doctrine of informed consent is part of English law." Summarising the decisions of the four of the five judges (including, of course, himself) in that case as "yes with reservations" he went on to look at the implications of "that very tentative move away from what some of us have seen as the predominance of power vested in the doctor."

What he said was that the "emotive term", "sovereignty" of the patient, had been reinstated and his statement of the law as he then saw it was encapsulated in the next two paragraphs: "So all the emotive phrase means is that the medical ethic must include not only advice as to what is medically appropriate for the patient in his situation but also respect by the doctor for the rights of the patient outside the field of medicine. And one of those rights is the right, in the light of all information available to him – family and business as well as medical – to make his own decision as to whether or not he will accept the treatment that is being proposed.

One can therefore say that English law has advanced to this position: that the patient has a right, if he is fit to receive the information, and if he desires to receive the information, to make his decision, his choice, on the basis of relevant information medical as well as other."

Both these judgments, and indeed Lord Scarman's article, vindicated AVMA's view that the Courts had been abrogating their duty to make a decision on the issue of consent and allowing that decision to be taken by doctors. In every other type of case the Courts would listen to the evidence and then decide what the correct position was. In medical negligence, however, they would leave the decision to a "responsible body of medical men". That might have been acceptable in the case of something as technical as a medical issue, (although AVMA long argued that even in relation to medical matters the Courts gave too much power to the doctors). But consent is not a medical issue. It is an issue of fact and common sense. And we could not understand why the judges were prepared to allow doctors to make the decision. One of our solicitors suggested, tongue in cheek, that the reason for this was that some judges in their autumn years would be more likely to require the services of a doctor. They therefore did not want to upset them! Seemingly that did not apply to the Lords Scarman and Bridge. Their judgements made it clear that, (at least in some cases according to Lord Bridge), the decision could not be handed over to the medical profession.

Although the patient lost her case, which was a tragedy for her, the remarks of such senior judges as Lords Scarman and Bridge, the careful analysis of the issue of consent in medical negligence cases and the massive publicity and interest aroused by the case had the same effect on the medical establishment as a successful claim would have done. Doctors soon began talking about "Informed Consent" as if it were something that was always required. In fact the medical profession has come to recognise that doctors have to give much more information to a patient to enable him or her to make an informed decision. Indeed, the version of the General Medical Council's publication "Seeking Consent: The ethical considerations" published in November 1998 underlines this:

> "Successful relationships between doctors and patients depend on trust. To establish that trust you must respect patients' autonomy – their right to decide whether or not to undergo any medical intervention even where a refusal may result in harm to themselves or in their own death. Patients must be given sufficient information, in a way that they can understand, to enable them to exercise their right to make informed decisions about their care."

In effect, the case of Sidaway brought patient safety and justice out of the shadows although there was and still is a long way to go.

By the time of the case of *Chester v Afshar [2004] UKHL 41; [2004] 4 All ER 587*, even the courts were accepting the doctrine of informed consent. This case revolved around a different but important issue but in dealing with that issue reference was made to the question of consent. The main issue was one of causation. In order to succeed in any personal injury case it is necessary to prove three things: firstly that the defendant was negligent, in other words in breach of duty, secondly that the negligence caused the injury and thirdly that the injury caused some loss which could be compensated. The issue of causation was, until this case, sacrosanct. To explain the implications of this case I can do no better than quote in full the Web entry from Charles Russell, the solicitors who acted for the complainant in that case:

> "**Modification of conventional causation principles to provide remedies where duty had been breached.** The strict requirement in tort that the Claimant prove that the

Defendant's negligence had caused the harm suffered was modified to permit a claim where a patient could not show that, had her surgeon complied with his duty to warn her of the risks of the surgery, she would never have consented to the operation.

Miss Chester had suffered repeated episodes of back pain. Between 1988 and 1994 this was treated conservatively through a course of injections. In 1994 Miss Chester was referred to Mr Afshar, a consultant neurosurgeon, who advised and performed surgery." [*I digress to comment that it is interesting to note that once again a neurosurgeon was involved. It is, or certainly was, well known among the medical profession that surgeons were less prone to communicate with their patients than other branches of the profession*]. "As a result of the surgery Miss Chester suffered the rare, but recognised, complication "cauda equina syndrome", causing partial paralysis. The operation was not performed negligently and there was nothing to suggest that the chances of the complication occurring, estimated at between 1–2%, were increased by the manner in which Mr Afshar performed the surgery.

The issue before the House of Lords was whether Mr Afshar was liable to Miss Chester for failing to warn her, prior to performing the operation, of the danger of the complication occurring. *One of the duties imposed on surgeons by the law of tort even prior to the case of Sidaway is to warn patients of the risks of any proposed surgery, so as to enable them to make an informed decision about whether to undergo that surgery – the doctrine of "informed consent".* [My italics.] It is accepted that, if a claimant can show that, had she been informed of the risks, she would not have consented to the surgery, the surgeon will be liable for any damage resulting from the realisation of those risks. The difficulty in this case was that Miss Chester was unable to show that knowledge of the risk would have altered her decision to consent to the operation – all that she could show was that it would have caused her to delay her decision, pending possible further opinions. As such, the conventional "but for" test applied in tortious cases was not satisfied: it could not be said that, but for Mr Afshar's failure to warn his patient of the risk, Miss Chester would not have consented to the operation and thus not have suffered the resulting damage. Nor could it be said that the risk was increased by the failure to warn: it existed as an inevitable risk of the operation, regardless of how skilfully the operation was performed.

The Lords held by a majority of three to two that, in order to do justice, conventional causation principles must be modified in the present case to allow the claim. Causation issues could not be separated from policy considerations: the function of the law was to enable rights to be vindicated and to provide remedies where duties had been breached. The injury suffered was within the scope of Mr Afshar's duty to warn. Mr Afshar had accordingly violated his patient's right to make an informed choice: Miss Chester could not be said to have given informed consent to the surgery "in the full legal sense".

The decision of the Lords to modify the tried and trusted causation test is a momentous one. The only parallel is the case *of Fairchild v Glenhaven Funeral Services Ltd [2003] 1 AC 32*, an asbestos case in which the test was modified to overcome the fact that the claimant employees could not prove which of their employers (all in breach of their duty to minimise the risks of exposure to asbestos dust) had been responsible for the actual exposure which resulted in the onset of mesothelioma. In *Chester v Afshar* the Lords recognised that such modifications were exceptional, but also that they could not be limited to a particular set of facts. However, *Chester* arguably represents a significant extension of the situations where the strict requirement to show causation will be overlooked: in *Fairchild* it was impossible to show which employer was actually responsible for the critical exposure – therefore causation could not be technically proved. On the facts of *Chester*, it would not be possible for a claimant to prove that, had she been warned of the dangers, she would definitely not have consented to the operation; the reason it could not be proven in *Chester* was because there was no conclusive evidence that the Claimant would have come to this decision."

For me, and others concerned with patient safety, what is so interesting about this case is that while the issue as to whether a claimant could claim damages when she could not show that had she been warned she would not have undergone the operation was hotly contested, the *need* to give her sufficient information to enable her to make a decision was taken as read. Informed consent had become enshrined in English law.

The other interesting aspect of this decision is the fact that it demonstrated how the courts were increasingly beginning to see medical negligence cases from the patient's point of view and were prepared to make new law to help them.

Important as these consent cases were, typically the media were far more interested in another milestone case decided in the same year as *Sidaway*, 1985, conducted by David Body because it dealt with the amount of compensation. Samir Aboul-Housn, a bright student aged 21 with a university career in front of him, was reduced to the mental age of 7 by a negligent medical mistake. In that case, against the Italian Hospital, for the first time damages of over £1m were awarded for a victim of a medical accident. The figure was an emotive one at that time and led to those who should have known better to beat the drum for containing damages for victims rather than urging greater safety in medicine. The media played much on that issue without making clear that only £85,000 of the award was for pain, suffering and loss of amenities – a pitifully small sum when one thinks about his suffering. The bulk of the award was simply compensating the young man for what he had actually lost in potential earnings plus the cost of caring for him for the rest of his life.

The real significance of the judgment was that Courts were beginning to recognise that in medical negligence, as in other personal injury cases, the loss to the victim needs to be properly compensated and medical negligence lawyers were gaining the experience to quantify that loss properly.

Unfortunately, in the case of *Gregg v Scott [2005] UKHL 2* the Court took a step backwards insofar as common sense decisions are concerned. This case involved the somewhat complex issue of loss of chance. That is, rather than a person wanting compensation for having lost something tangible – money, their health etc. – they want it for having lost the chance, either of acquiring some benefit or avoiding some disadvantage. There had previously been a case in medical negligence involving the question of loss of chance but the House of Lords had not been prepared to answer the question whether loss of a chance is compensable damage in the context of clinical negligence claims (*Hotson v East Berkshire Health Authority [1987] AC 750*).

In *Gregg* the House of Lords did answer it by deciding that where a claimant has suffered a loss of a chance of recovery as a result of medical negligence, but the chance is less than even, he or she is not entitled to compensation for that lost chance. That decision in my view, and that of many others, goes against common sense. As the barrister, Charles Foster of Outer Temple Chambers, says in an article on the case to be found on the Web, "Imagine that a patient has cancer. He goes to his doctor at a stage when he has a 45% chance of recovery. The doctor negligently says that the condition is benign. The necessary treatment is delayed for months. When the correct diagnosis is finally made the prospects of recovery are nil. Should the diminished chance of recovery not sound in damages? "

Fortunately, as Charles Foster went on to point out, in *Chester* one of the Law Lords, Lady Hale, made it clear that in certain circumstances it would be possible to claim compensation for loss of chance although describing it in a somewhat different way. She said that on conventional principles, that is, not on the basis of loss of chance, the defendant is liable for any *extra* pain, suffering, loss of amenity, financial loss and loss of expectation of life which may have resulted from the delay. If, without the delay, the claimant would have achieved a longer gap before more radical treatment became necessary, then he should be entitled to damages to reflect the acceleration in his suffering. If the pain and suffering he would have suffered anyway was made worse by the anguish of knowing that his disease could have been detected earlier, then he should be compensated for that. Furthermore, she said that there is also the distinct possibility that the delay reduced Mr Gregg's life expectancy in that had he been treated when he should have been treated, his median life expectancy then would have been x years, whereas given the delay in treatment his median life expectancy from then is x minus y. There might therefore be a modest claim in respect of the "lost years".

I have not rehearsed the full argument that Charles Foster set out, still less the whole of the judgments, but simply sufficient to show that the Courts are not inexorably moving in favour of fairness for patients, as well as to show that hopefully the issue of loss of chance is not dead.

One of the cruelest legal principles, as far as people who suffer medical negligence are concerned, is that of limitation. As the word suggests it refers to limiting the circumstances in which a claim can be brought. Insofar as personal injury claims are concerned The Limitation Act 1980 deals with the time within which a claim for personal injury must be brought. The Act provides that a claim must be brought within three years of the injury or within three years of the injured person having knowledge of the injury. Section 14 of the Act defines the date of knowledge as the date on which the claimant first had knowledge of the following facts:

(a)   That the injury is significant
(b)   That it is attributable in whole or in part to the act or omission
(c)   The identity of the defendant

It also goes on to say that knowledge that any acts or omissions did or did not, as a matter of law, involve negligence, nuisance or breach of duty is irrelevant. In other words, if a person does not take action within the limitation period he or she cannot argue later, when perhaps at a social gathering, a lawyer tells them that they could have sued, that they did not know that what had been done was negligent, nuisance or a breach of duty.

Insofar as "ordinary" personal injury is concerned in the main that is not a problem. If a person is in a car accident or falls off a ladder at work they will usually know when they were injured, the nature of their injury and who had caused it or if someone is to blame. There are of course obvious exceptions where, for example, the injured person is in a coma or has some brain injury which prevents them being aware of what has happened. In those latter circumstances the court would extend the limitation period beyond three years.

Medical negligence injuries are more complex and there has been a lot of litigation about the question of when a person acquires the knowledge as defined above. One of the court decisions that really made me angry was that in the case of *Dobbie v Medway Health Authority (1994) 1 WLR 1234.* In April 1973 Mrs Dobbie was admitted to hospital for a biopsy of a lump in her breast. Without further consent the surgeon removed her breast because in the course of the operation he decided that the lump appeared malignant. Subsequently, however, a pathologist's report revealed that the lump had been benign.

Mrs Dobbie, although obviously upset, did not realise that anything wrong had been done to her. How would she if the doctors did not explain? However, in 1988 she read a report of a similar case in which a woman had obtained compensation. So she consulted solicitors who began proceedings on her behalf by issuing a writ in 1989. This was of course 16 years after the operation and the solicitors for the hospital naturally claimed that she was too late to bring the claim as she was outside the limitation period. Her solicitors argued that she should have the benefit of the exceptions to the time limit in that she did not have the requisite knowledge under the Limitation Act.

What Mrs Dobbie said in evidence is in my view of great significance: "After the operation I, of course, knew that my breast had been removed but having been told that when the surgeon opened me up it had looked suspicious I accepted it was safer to remove the breast in case the lump was cancerous. As far as I was concerned the surgeon had acted in my best interest and had acted perfectly properly... I had no reason to question the surgeon's wisdom or judgment. I was told that the lump in the breast was benign and that I should be grateful that I did not have cancer."

Once more I must digress to comment on this last sentence. For many years after AVMA was founded doctors would continue to regard a patient as ungrateful if, the original problem having been cured, the patient complained that in curing the problem the doctor had negligently left the patient with, for example, a disability with which he or she should not have been left. They should be grateful that the major problem had been cured and not worry that the result was less than perfect because of the doctor's negligence. Happily it is unlikely that a doctor would suggest that today although I have no doubt that such feelings are still nurtured.

In Mrs Dobbie's case the Judge held that she did have the necessary knowledge and could therefore not proceed with her case. But worse was to come. The Limitation Act also provides that even if the claimant did have the knowledge the Judge can exercise his or her discretion to allow the case to go forward if that is fair. What the Judge said in Mrs Dobbie's case was that because she knew she had had a breast wrongly removed she should have made enquiries and he therefore refused to exercise his discretion.

The comments I made in the *AVMA Medical and Legal Journal Spring 1994* are just as relevant today – "I find it difficult to believe that any intelligent person would expect an ordinary patient, certainly in 1976 [sic] to realise in those circumstances that she had suffered an injury."

I have dealt with all these cases in some detail in order to demonstrate two things. Firstly to show that, from being an area of the law that was swept up into the ordinary law of personal injury and therefore virtually ignored, medical negligence has become a definitive branch of the law which has led to complex and ground-breaking litigation. Secondly to show that the expertise of lawyers in this area has had a major impact in ensuring that victims of medical accidents secure what they are entitled to and in doing so have advanced patient safety. AVMA has had no small part to play in these achievements. Although these cases are, for the lay reader, somewhat technical, what all of them have in common is that as a result of the work AVMA has done over the years judges are prepared to discuss the law of medical negligence in the context of patients' rights and needs. Although all that they can do in the end is award financial compensation, the effect of their decisions is that patient safety is enhanced.

# Chapter 8
# The response of the health carers

All of us at AVMA had hoped that highlighting the problem of medical accidents would be of benefit to patients, health carers and the government. All of these would benefit if the obvious response were adopted, namely to stop, or at least dramatically reduce, the number and seriousness of the accidents. Patients would obviously benefit because patient safety would be improved and fewer of them would suffer unnecessary damage; doctors would benefit because fewer of them would suffer the trauma of injuring a patient whom they had intended to help or of being at the wrong end of soul-destroying litigation; and the government and health care providers would benefit by an enormous saving of the costs of compensation, additional treatment and care and litigation.

As far as the government was concerned, in the first few years it appeared to have no interest in the problem whatsoever. The health carers on the other hand responded to meet what they saw as simply a financial problem with a two-pronged attack – defensive medicine and no fault compensation.

Defensive medicine was bubbling up as an issue long before AVMA was founded, particularly in the United States. In a (draft) 1986 article by Iain Chalmers, now Sir Iain, he referred to a survey by the American College of Obstetricians and Gynaecologists. It reported that in the previous five years the frequency of lawsuits involving obstetricians had tripled and in New York half the obstetricians had been sued on more than one occasion. He went on to write that "The most frequently reported changes in obstetric practice resulting from this epidemic of litigation are increased testing, increased documentation, increased monitoring in labour, increased use of caesarean sections and refusal to take on 'high risk' cases for care."

The interesting thing is that apart from the last-mentioned, all the consequences would appear to be good and in the interests of patient safety. It was argued however, that in fact these additional procedures were unnecessary and were only being adopted because of the threat of litigation.

That was the American scene at the time. Of course that scene was not a little influenced by the fact that in the United States medicine is a commercial exercise.

In the UK the first major litigation influence on obstetric practice was the decision in the case of *Whitehouse v Jordan [1981 AER 267]*. In that case an obstetrician was sued because a baby had suffered brain damage. In 1978 the trial Court found that he had been negligent because he had "pulled too long and too hard" in his attempt to deliver a baby vaginally, with forceps, before resorting to caesarean delivery. Although the Appeal Court, and subsequently the House of Lords reversed the decision, among the obstetric fraternity the damage had been done. Between 1978 and 1979 there was a dramatic fall in the forceps delivery rate and the largest ever annual increase in the caesarean section rate. (Office for Population Censuses and Surveys, 1984.) Ironically, for the obstetrician the result in the first court was not all bad although of course he did suffer personally from having been criticised by the court as well as having to wait years before his name was cleared to his personal satisfaction. However, from his practice's point of view, as I was told by a number of other obstetricians, he found that after the media report of the trial his private obstetric practice increased substantially – name recognition is all!

Clearly obstetricians were beginning to practise defensive medicine although at that time there was little use of the term. When AVMA's work began to have results in the litigation field, and not only were successful obstetric claims becoming more frequent but the awards of compensation were following the lead of the million pound award in the *Aboul-Housn* case, the issue of defensive medicine came to the fore. Articles, letters and lectures began to appear with increasing regularity on the subject. The thrust was always that litigation was causing obstetricians to carry out unnecessary caesarean sections. There were even suggestions from senior obstetricians that medical students were not choosing to go into obstetrics and there would soon be no obstetricians left.

These pronouncements were beginning to sound like a threat to the public – "if you don't stop suing us we won't provide you with obstetricians!"

In another draft article by Iain Chalmers in 1986 entitled "The Growth of Defensive Obstetric Practice in Britain: a Cause for Concern" he wrote that "as a consequence British obstetricians are now often putting legal considerations before medical considerations in their clinical practice." It was obvious that that was exactly what they were doing. They were openly stating that, because of the fear of litigation, they were carrying out more caesarean sections. I had many battles with obstetricians on those issues both in private and on public platforms when I drew this to their attention. AVMA's view was always that defensive medicine was not an option for obstetricians. In the interests of their patients they had to practise good medicine. If we look at the quotation from the American College of Obstetricians and Gynaecologists to which I have referred it seems to me that litigation was having a number of beneficial effects – "increased testing, increased documentation, increased monitoring in labour".

And it was not only in obstetrics that this paranoia was beginning to operate. The issue became such a hot one that BBC Newsnight picked it up in a programme on the 21st October 1986. On that programme, Robert Atlay, the then Secretary of the Royal College of Obstetricians and Gynaecologists (RCOG) said: "Why then, are we going through all this hassle of all the explanations and all the trouble we are going to – because we do not want to end up in court fighting our patients because we didn't give them proper explanations." (Transcript of the programme)

Also on that programme Mervyn Kidd, another obstetrician, when talking about the caesarean rate said: "one is perhaps stepping that little bit outside what is accepted practice." It was a measure of AVMA's growing importance that I was invited to appear on the programme as well – fortunately it was before the days of Jeremy Paxman because the programme was definitely on the side of the doctors! As I said on that programme, AVMA's attitude was that "if a doctor carries out a procedure because he or she thinks that will avoid litigation if something goes wrong, that is appalling."

I was so concerned about how this practice of "defensive" medicine was developing that I wrote to Sir John Walton, the President of the General Medical Council, asking whether the behaviour admitted by these consultants might amount to professional misconduct. After having to write again following a mealy-mouthed reply from someone on behalf of the President I received the following reply which I believe vindicated AVMA's stance:

> "The President has carefully considered your letter and has noted your further comments regarding so-called 'defensive medicine'. He has asked me to assure you that if the Council were to receive a complaint, supported by evidence, that a doctor had in a specific case jeopardized the welfare of a particular patient by subordinating the patient's best medical interests to other extraneous considerations, he would regard such an allegation as a very serious matter, and would consider whether the circumstances of the case and the evidence available might justify the institution of disciplinary proceedings against the doctor concerned, on the grounds that the doctor had seriously neglected his professional duty towards a patient."

I publicised this wherever and whenever I could and particularly whenever I had the ear of obstetricians. I also pointed out that in practising so-called defensive medicine doctors were laying themselves open not only to disciplinary action but also to litigation. One of the examples I used was in relation to caesarean sections themselves. If a doctor carried out an unnecessary section and then something went wrong during that operation the mother or child might have a claim even if no negligence in the operation was involved. The plaintiff could argue that the doctor should not have carried out the caesarean in the first place. Neither the GMC President's warning nor my examples ended the doctors' campaign. In particular the then President of the RCOG continued to maintain that obstetrics was being adversely affected by the amount of litigation against obstetricians. Slowly, however, the force of this attack began to abate as a result of the repeated exposure of its contradictions. Less was seen in the media and eventually that same president said to me that he could "live with the position". (Personal conversation)

Nevertheless the concept of defensive medicine continued to bedevil the issue of medical accidents and prevent the medical profession from addressing the problem of medical accidents objectively. Interestingly it was a public health doctor who exposed the real myth of defensive medicine. In January 1995 Nicholas Summerton of Bradford Health Authority's department of public health medicine published a study on the subject in the *British Medical Journal* [BMJ 1995; 310:27-29]. Writing in the *Guardian* on the 7th January 1995 Chris Mihill showed how Dr Summerton demonstrated that "doctors who carry out extra tests on patients in case they are sued may be giving the public a better service than those who do not."

"In a new survey," wrote Chris Mihill, "Nicholas Summerton ... says defensive medicine – particularly more detailed explanations of what is to be done and more extensive note-taking of symptoms – can benefit patients. Dr Summerton asked 300 general practitioners whether they had changed the way they worked for fear of complaints or legal action. Ninety-eight per cent said that they had made some practice changes in case a patient complained. Around 60% of the doctors said they were offering diagnostic testing, more referrals to hospital, increased follow-ups and more detailed explanations. Some 40% said they would avoid treating certain conditions in the surgery, and a similar proportion said they would consider extra diagnostic tests even where there was some risk to the patient. Nearly 30% said they would consider prescribing unnecessary drugs. Nine out of ten of the doctors said they took more detailed notes and gave patients more detailed explanations, and a third said they did more screening work or undertook practice audits to improve what they were doing. Dr Summerton said, 'Some defensive practices, such as more detailed note-taking, are clearly beneficial, but others will have adverse effects on both patient care and resource allocation. The existence of negative defensive medicine is best viewed as a symptom of the fundamental problems inherent within the present regulatory systems."

What comes across absolutely clearly is that most doctors simply do not understand the implications of so-called defensive medicine. Taking more detailed notes and giving more detailed explanations is clearly in the interest of the patient and is good medicine. But for doctors to admit that they give *unnecessary* drugs demonstrates what I explained before: that doctors can actually get into more trouble by practising what they understand as defensive medicine rather than good medicine.

Defensive medicine was however, only one of the tools utilised by the medical profession in trying to stop litigation. What disturbed us at AVMA was the way the profession appeared to be turning a blind eye to the most obvious answer and the one which was most patient-centred, namely reducing the number of accidents. Instead they looked only at solutions that might get doctors off the hook. In addition to claims about defensive medicine the solution which they found most attractive was what was called, in shorthand, no fault compensation. A system, in other words, that does not look at whether an injury has been caused by anyone's negligence, but simply compensates a patient for any injury that is caused during medical care. On the face of it this does sound an extremely attractive solution. And I have no doubt many doctors were ardent protagonists because they genuinely believed it would be to patients' advantage. The argument most used by the BMA went like this: There could be three patients lying side by side suffering with brain damage. The first who had suffered as a result of provable medical negligence might end up receiving compensation from the Court amounting to millions of pounds; the second who had suffered as a result of the whooping cough vaccine would receive statutory compensation which at that time was £20,000; the third with no identifiable culpable cause would receive no compensation at all.

They argued, with justification, that such a system was wholly unjust. They and the medical profession generally referred to the systems in Sweden and New Zealand which were forms of no fault compensation which in their view were much fairer and were operating successfully. There were, however, major downsides to those systems and the only definite advantage was from the doctors' point of view in that they resulted in doctors no longer being sued for negligence. In any event those systems compensate the first two examples but only the third if it could be shown there was an "accident" as such.

It is not the place in this book to discuss the issue of no fault compensation in detail. It has been debated over many years and numerous articles, learned and not so learned, have been written on the topic. However, it is interesting to note what Peter Ransley said about it in the introduction to AVMA's first Annual Report in 1983, when he highlighted this issue which AVMA would have to face throughout the time that I led it: "An answer that is going to come up more and more in 1984 is the concept of no fault compensation. Under this a victim does not have to prove negligence. He is automatically compensated by the state. It sounds fine. The medical profession is likely to welcome it because it does away with the threat of doctors being dragged through the courts. Most victims would be compensated, instead of the few that win at judicial roulette. Why then should we be cautious? Because we fear that compensation levels would be low and in many cases inadequate. Because on their past record there is no sign that the doctors will accept an enquiry system that will disclose to victims what happened to them."

Suffice now to give an outline of why AVMA was so set against it and why I say the medical profession wanted to use it as a tool to get doctors off the hook.

In February 1991 the MP Rosie Barnes presented a Bill to Parliament entitled National Health Service (Compensation) Bill. This attempted to introduce a system which would compensate victims of medical accidents without the need for litigation. In an article setting out AVMA's comments on the Bill, I summarised our arguments against no fault compensation. I can do no better than quote from it. First I established what we understood that patients wanted (and I believe still want) when things go wrong based on the evidence of the thousands of unhappy patients who had sought our help over the years:

> "The primary mischief to be addressed by any legislation to put victims of medical accidents in a better position than they are now is the lack of accountability of the Health Care professionals for those accidents. What patients need above all when things go wrong is to know that they have gone wrong and not to be told that they have simply been the victim of a disease or the usual complications of an operation; they need to know why they went wrong; they

need to have a full and meaningful apology; they need to know that other health carers will be told and understand what went wrong and, using that knowledge will do everything they can to put things right; and they need to know what action will be taken whether with regard to individuals or systems, to ensure that similar accidents do not happen to other patients in the future. In addition, many of them will need financial compensation to maintain or rebuild their shattered lives."

I made it clear that:

"Any scheme that concentrates overwhelmingly on the compensation aspect as the present Bill does and fails to give at least equal but preferably greater attention to these matters will not deal with the mischief that causes the greatest distress to thousands of victims of medical accidents."

Further:

"What must be recognised is the control which the health care professionals, and doctors in particular, have exercised until recently in ensuring that the needs of victims are not recognised. By sticking together, by controlling the knowledge about medical matters and by creating an aura of inviolability around themselves, and by consciously or subconsciously working on the fears of people about health and life and death they made it quite impossible for any of them to be brought to account for their actions."

I also made it clear that AVMA did not wish to defend the legal system. Having had contact with thousands of victims of medical accidents AVMA was more aware than most people of the defects of the system. However, I went on:

"One matter is overlooked by those who would bring about change; the legal system does ensure that in a large number of cases the issues are properly examined; it is the only system that exercises any real kind of accountability over health care professionals; it does, for those who qualify for its help, deal with all the needs of victims of medical accidents – for compensation, for explanations and for ensuring that bad practices are highlighted and therefore changed so that similar accidents do not happen again."

I might have added that sometimes they even received an apology as a result of the litigation.

And so we came to the conclusion that:

> "Before that is changed it is essential that a new system is devised that does not throw away the hard-won gains provided by the legal system. Any Bill that is proposed to change the system root and branch must be a patients' Bill."

We therefore objected to the Bill on the basis, amongst other reasons, that it:

> "displays the lack of understanding of the real needs of victims and the ways in which the health care professionals have denied and deny those needs and it therefore fails to provide patients with essential protection."

AVMA had been putting forward these arguments for years. The medical profession did not want to listen. Their representatives, and particularly the defence organisations, continually expressed surprise that an organisation that represented patients who had suffered did not support proposals for no fault compensation. But that was the whole point. With our experience of nearly a hundred thousand patients we could not support such a system, for the reasons I have explained. Yet the medical profession did not appear to ask themselves the question, why is that, and so they remained oblivious to the answer. And that is why I say, and said repeatedly, that they, or at least those of most influence, appeared to see no fault compensation as a system to get them off the hook.

Like the doctors, Rosie Barnes also refused to listen to us though I met her on a number of occasions before the terms of the Bill were finalised. She refused to make what we regarded as essential amendments to the Bill although she made a few minor ones as a result of our conversations. Consequently we briefed MPs and Lords to oppose the Bill. Many other patients' organisations, including the Association of Community Health Councils did so as well. The Bill did not pass. I do not suggest that it was solely because of AVMA's opposition that the Bill failed. But I do think that if AVMA had campaigned strongly for the Bill then MPs would have found it harder to resist taking on board the views of the only organisation thoroughly versed in the needs of victims of medical accidents. This would have been reinforced if AVMA and the BMA had mounted a joint campaign.

The campaign of the medical profession for a system of no fault compensation was so effective that not only did it influence MPs like Rosie Barnes but even Des Wilson, one of the founders of Shelter and a campaigner for citizens' rights, took up the cudgels. He established an organisation called Citizen Action Compensation Campaign. Notwithstanding the name the campaign was not directed to compensation across the board but only to compensation in medical accidents for which he advocated a system of no fault compensation. Once again the views of AVMA were ignored. I questioned at the time why Wilson should target medical accidents where the largest guesstimates (those made by AVMA) were indicating a possible total of 50,000 accidents a year compared with industrial accidents of 147,000 a year and road traffic accidents of 239,000 a year. But of course Wilson was a great publicist and medical accidents were a hot topic. (It is an irony that when, many years later, a proper analysis of medical accidents was made, it was discovered that there were likely to be more than a million such accidents a year, rather than the 50,000 that AVMA was estimating in 1989. (Organisation With a Memory, OWAM, Department of Health June 2000 – see below.)

We realised at AVMA that in the face of such a populist campaign it was not enough for AVMA simply to advance arguments, some of them quite complex, as to why such a system was inappropriate for medical accidents. It was essential that we put forward a positive solution with a description as accessible as no fault compensation. Previously, having summarised all the arguments against no fault, we had come up with the idea of "Accountable Compensation". This had gained some publicity and the LAG (Legal Action Group) Bulletin of May 1989 ran an article under that title. However, that was not enough to set against Rosie Barnes' Bill. Indeed, although ACHCEW, the Association of Community Health Councils in England & Wales, agreed with us that the Bill should be opposed, Toby Harris, Secretary of ACHCEW, made it quite clear that unless we were able to come up with an alternative proposal simple opposition would be ineffective. He and I then produced a proposal for a Health Standards Inspectorate which was finally published by our two organisations jointly in November 1991.

The essential thrust of this proposal, unlike any other form of No Fault scheme or proposal, aimed to deal with the issue of medical accidents in a comprehensive way. Because of AVMA's experience over ten years in dealing directly with over 100,000 patients who had been or believed themselves to have been victims of a medical accident, plus CHCs' experience with many more complainants, we were better able than anyone to understand what patients or their relatives required when something went wrong. The Inspectorate proposal made it clear that:

> "8.3  These concerns of patients can be expressed more formally as issues which must be dealt with by any system which seeks to provide justice for victims of medical accidents as follows:
>
> (i)    Standards
>
> (ii)   Explanations
>
> (iii)  Accountability
>
> (iv)   Compensation

The proposal carefully analysed the various no fault schemes in existence at the time. It showed that they did not deal with standards or accountability and that in both the Swedish and New Zealand schemes the issue of fault still had to be addressed albeit in another guise. Under the Swedish system compensation was only paid if an accident was "avoidable" so the question would always arise as to how to say whether an accident was avoidable. Under the New Zealand scheme, compensation would only be paid if there had been personal injury by accident. Whether there had been an accident would also revolve around the issue of fault. The AVMA/ACHCEW scheme therefore proposed a Health Inspectorate and Complaints authority which would be able to deal with all the above issues.

Of course we cannot claim the credit on our own for ensuring that a full-scale no fault compensation system was not introduced at that time but our arguments did strongly influence the debate.

Although I have dealt at some length with the very negative response of the health carers towards the successful growth of AVMA there were positive responses as well. I have already mentioned the way in which doctors started coming forward to give expert evidence for patients. Emboldened by this we decided quite early on to try to get doctors more involved in the general work of AVMA, particularly on the patient safety side. We already had a budding (and, for AVMA, very remunerative) Lawyers' Support Group and this, coupled with the increasing amount of medical negligence litigation, resulted in the public, the medical profession, the media and the policy makers perceiving us as primarily interested in litigation. Indeed, even some organisations that had considerable contact with AVMA continued over the years to believe that our only interest was litigation. Even in the late nineties someone like Roger Goss, who worked for the Patients' Association and later founded an organisation called Patient Concern, was surprised when I pointed out to him that litigation was a minor part of AVMA's work.

So as early as 1983 I decided to set up a Doctors' Support Group. The idea was initially to have a small group of doctors already committed to the aims of AVMA to discuss ideas and how to involve more doctors. As with the Lawyers' Support Group the name implied both support by doctors for AVMA and support by AVMA for doctors. Thus the agenda for the first meeting on the 14th November 1983 included –

"A.  To support AVMA in its work. This will involve consideration of the following topics:

(ii)  Ethics involved. Problems over second opinions and expert opinions"

And

"B.  To help change the attitudes of doctors toward accidents and negligence. This would involve:

(i)  Consideration of the effect on a doctor and his/her career of both "accidents" and negligence."

Although the meetings we held were extremely useful and not only led to the recruitment of more sympathetic doctors, mainly as medical experts, but also gave me insights into the approach of the medical profession to the issue, the Group did not thrive.

It was probably premature, as were the two further attempts to establish a group in 1985 and 1988. The problem was that unlike with the lawyers, we did not really have anything to offer doctors other than the satisfaction of changing attitudes in their profession. I was certainly unable at that stage to get across the concept that helping victims of medical accidents and approaching them sympathetically was actually part of a doctor's duty of care. It was not until the 1998 edition of *Good Medical Practice*, the doctors' bible, that such a concept was touched upon: (paragraph 17):

> "If a patient under your care has suffered serious harm, through misadventure or for any other reason, you should act immediately to put matters right, if that is possible. You should explain fully to the patient what has happened and the likely long-and short-term effects. When appropriate you should offer an apology."

It was clarified and strengthened in the 2006 edition where, most importantly, the following were some of the words added (paragraph 31):

> "You must not allow a patient's complaint to affect adversely the care or treatment you provide or arrange."

These words were of crucial importance because one of AVMA's major complaints over the years had been that in covering up what had gone wrong doctors were often unable to give the patient the necessary remedial treatment for fear that that would expose the wrongdoing.

# Chapter 9
# Casework – working with victims

At the heart of AVMA's work from its inception was the help we gave or tried to give to those who had suffered or believed they had suffered what we chose to call a medical accident. There have been over the years numerous misconceptions about AVMA's role and many of these arose from the interpretation different people put on the term "medical accident". From time to time, almost throughout my tenure as AVMA's Chief Executive, I had a number of interesting but somewhat arcane discussions with Roy Palmer, then Secretary of the Medical Protection Society, about this issue. Given his position and his brief to defend his members, and perhaps the medical profession generally, against claims for negligence, it seemed important to him to challenge me on the definition. Similarly, as recently as 2008, I found myself omitted by the Appointments Commission from a shortlist on an application for a Board position on a health quango on the grounds that my history showed that I was mostly concerned with medical negligence and compensation.

That is why I refer to the fact that we "chose" to refer to medical accidents. For us the term was quite clear and whilst it encompassed negligence it in no way referred only to blameworthy actions or omissions amenable to claims for compensation. Indeed, while it has to be acknowledged that AVMA made its name through its high-profile work in the legal arena our main concern was patient safety, that is, that accidents should not happen. Although the origin of the organisation was a television play that dealt with negligence and compensation, we recognised from our steering group days that when something went wrong during medical care the patient or their relative was concerned initially about the *fact* that something had gone wrong and the patient was suffering. The questions as to why it went wrong and whether someone was to blame were ancillary matters to be dealt with at some other time. So from the outset, when someone approached us with a problem which had arisen during medical care we saw it as our role, not immediately to try and define whether there had been a blameworthy event, but to help the client to deal with the problem as he or she saw it and to alleviate their distress if we could.

Our experience with clients over the years reinforced our view that compensation was not the primary aim of those who believed they had suffered a medical accident. What they want first and foremost is an explanation. This is now commonplace among those helping people who have suffered a medical accident and among Government; but it was not always so. It was as a result of AVMA's experience with thousands of clients, and repeatedly making the point clear, that it became accepted. Indeed, whenever I had the opportunity, whether in addressing conferences, meeting with government Ministers or speaking to the media I advanced what we came to refer to as AVMA's mantra: that what victims wanted was justice which we interpreted as: an explanation of what happened and why, a meaningful apology, treatment to put right what had gone wrong if that were possible, that steps should be taken to ensure that what had happened to them should not happen to anyone else and last of all, compensation.

Of course, a major part of our work was "political" because we very soon identified the main issue as being one of patient safety. That meant working to change the culture of the health carers and the attitude of government in order to ensure that wherever possible accidents did not happen. That is where our work for clients had a dual purpose. Not only did we have a role to help individuals but the fact that we worked at the coal face with those who had suffered gave us both an insight into what was needed as well as the authority to speak for change. Time and again a particular case, or a group of cases, would expose what we considered a scandal and I would use those cases to berate the health carers and endeavour to bring about change in the interests of patient safety.

The main thrust of AVMA's work on patient safety in the early days was to try to make healthcare professionals learn from their mistakes. The problem was, however, that before you can learn from mistakes you have to acknowledge them. And that was the most difficult thing to get health carers to do. At the hospital level we were dealing with a huge bureaucracy and it often seemed to us that hospitals treated complaints according to a formula, regarding the complainant as a nuisance to be got rid of as quickly and painlessly as possible. What upset complainants, and absolutely infuriated me, were the lengths to which hospital employees, whether complaints officers or indeed the Chief Executive, would go in order to avoid apologising, making any admission, or paying compensation.

In trying to deal with complaints in the early days of AVMA I was reminded of a joke that appeared to encapsulate the attitudes of the hospital authorities. A man was travelling on an overnight sleeper from London to Glasgow. Throughout the night he was plagued by fleabites and was unable to sleep. He was horrified when he switched on the light at one stage to see that his cabin was in fact infested with fleas. The next day he dashed off a furious letter of complaint to the train company. After only a couple of days he received a reply from no less than the Chief Executive of the company. He was profusely apologetic if not grovelling. He explained that the company maintained the highest standards of cleanliness and had never had such a complaint before. Nevertheless he had arranged for all his company's coaches to be fumigated, the offending coach would be renovated from top to toe and those responsible for cleaning trains would be disciplined.

Without doubt, such a letter would have satisfied the complainant. Unfortunately, however, attached to the letter by a paperclip was a note in handwriting: "Gladys – send the usual flea letter."

Thus the typical letter from a Chief Executive back in the 80s would begin "I am sorry that you feel that the hospital has not provided you with an adequate service." As far as the hospital was concerned, because they used the word "sorry" they were apologising. Of course anyone could see that they were not apologising for what had happened, or what they had done, but simply because the complainant "felt" let down. Not for the fact that he or she had been let down. When I had seen this formula used time and again by Chief Executives all over the country it became obvious that it was indeed a formula and they knew exactly what they were doing. Because we had the evidence we were able to expose this and after a time, perhaps two years, that particular offensive construction was abandoned.

However, the hospitals, and indeed doctors, continued to be terrified lest an apology were seen as an admission of liability leading to virtually automatic compensation. The Defence organisations, and particularly the Medical Defence Union, always claimed when I confronted them, that they advised their members that an apology was not an admission of liability and an apology should always be given when appropriate. I saw their literature which purported to do that. Either it simply was not clear enough or when a doctor sought advice over a specific issue they received a different message. The proof of the pudding was in the eating – whenever I spoke to doctors they were adamant that their defence organisation advised them not to apologise.

A striking example of how I used the work we did with victims was the talk I gave to the Royal Postgraduate Medical School in 1991. I was able to identify for the audience of doctors how the medical profession, wittingly or unwittingly, was acting against the very people they should have been helping. Interestingly, it was the Medical School that chose the title for my talk, "Storming Kafka's Castle". It was nine years after AVMA was founded. Yet doctors still, rightly, regarded our attempts to bring justice to victims of medical accidents as Kafkaesque. This was because AVMA looked at the problem as being one of patient safety, justice and accountability, whilst doctors appeared to see the slow empowerment of patients as a threat, both to their reputations and their pockets. As a consequence, every step forward AVMA made in making it easier for victims to get explanations, accountability, compensation or simply an apology, was met by the health carers trying to make it more difficult.

To demonstrate this I can do no better than quote extensively from my own lecture. I make no apology for this because it is contemporaneous and shows just what the situation was for victims of medical accidents at that time and how AVMA was trying to persuade doctors to change their approach.

"If you look at the campaign by the healthcare professionals on medical accidents you see that it has at least four strands. The first is that too much litigation is causing defensive medicine; the second is that the way to deal with claims for compensation is by a scheme of 'no fault' compensation; the third is by risk management and 'secret' reporting of accidents; and the fourth is by reducing or removing the largest claims by making it impossible to prove that cerebral palsy is, in fact, caused by hypoxia at childbirth.

"Now, I am not challenging the bona fides of the vast majority of health care professionals who genuinely believe in each one of the four points and do not in any sense see them as a campaign to cause problems for victims seeking justice." [Note how I had to pussyfoot at the time!] "Nevertheless if we analyse each one in turn we see that there are hidden agendas in all of them. When we look at them together we see that the effect of each one separately, and all of them together, actually amount to a massive threat to victims being able to secure justice. We then see that from the patients' point of view this is just another way in which the large gains made by patients are to be clawed back.

"Insofar as defensive medicine is concerned, this is something created by the medical establishment to frighten patients off from taking legal action and which has now seeped into the psyche of medical practitioners. I was deeply disappointed to see that even the Government Chief Medical Officer gave credence to it in his address to the Royal College of Midwives."

I then dealt with the criticisms of defensive medicine and then simply touched on No Fault Compensation:

"I clearly cannot deal with the whole issue of 'no-fault' compensation. I have just mentioned it here because it is something being pushed by many members of the medical profession and in particular the BMA. But it is significant that it is rejected by AVMA, the only organisation representing victims of medical accidents because the way it is being proposed will make it even more difficult for patients to find out what really happened to them and to ensure some measure of accountability."

The third threat I dealt with was Risk Management which was just being introduced at that time (1991):

> "I must admit that when I first came across the concept, no doubt like many of you I welcomed it because it seemed to me that if you identified the risk of accidents you would reduce their number. I thought, therefore, that risk management referred to standards. As AVMA believes that the real and only answer to the growth in litigation is raising standards and reducing accidents, we thought we had common ground with those advocating risk management. Unless as much effort is placed on risk management as on claims management the latter will turn out to be another turn of the Kafkaesque screw, if I can risk mixing my metaphors. I would refer you to the booklet for managers called 'Quality Counts' by Brian Capstick already referred to (by other speakers) at length. He makes it quite clear that managing claims means dealing with accidents which happen, not with trying to reduce those accidents, but he doesn't differentiate between managing claims and risk save to say he is not concerned with risk. In case this comes as as big a shock to you as it did to me, let me quote from the relevant passages in the booklet:

>> 'An ongoing audit will also help to identify the factors that give rise to claims. They in turn will provide a basis for the development of measures to cut down the number of accidents that bring about claims in the first place.' [So far so good] However, …Managers should not expect short term financial benefits from programmes designed to help avoid medical errors…

>> Although there is a role for Managers to help with the identification of problem areas, the place to begin saving money is with the better management of accidents, untoward incidents and claims.'

> "So you see, he does not want managers to concentrate on avoiding accidents, but on saving money.

"Now I'm not suggesting that claims management was ever put forward by Brian Capstick, or anyone else for that matter, as a means of reducing accidents but I think patients could certainly have been forgiven if they had expected that this would be at least an equal concern of managers with saving money. And if you then add to that, the contention put forward by Mr Capstick elsewhere, that investigation into accidents should be secret to encourage personnel to be open about it, you can perhaps begin to see why, if there is no actual conspiracy to deny patients information, the effect of what is being proposed is something straight out of Kafka."

Finally I dealt with the issue of cerebral palsy:

"Now I would like to turn to the last point I have listed in the campaign against victims by health care professionals. Rather than starting with an analysis of what is happening let me start at the wrong end, as it were, and look at the effect of what is being argued. If it were right, as David Hall says," [David Hall was an earlier lecturer at the conference] that the number of cases of cerebral palsy caused by hypoxia is insignificant, or as suggested by others that whilst there is a small percentage it is not really possible to prove in most of those cases whether the cerebral palsy was caused by hypoxia or not, then victims, their parents, their families will not be able to get the money they need to give them some sort of reasonable existence. The patients will have been defeated. Will that produce three cheers from the professionals? Make no mistake, 'no-fault' compensation will not step into the breach. It will not give them any money. In every scheme so far invented it is necessary to show that a person has had an accident not simply that there was some, for example, congenital defect, before you get compensation. Without that requirement, we would still be talking about extended State benefits and, in fairness, that would have to apply to anyone with any kind of congenital defect. So unless you can prove that the cerebral palsy was caused by something going wrong – whether through negligence or not – these children will get nothing.

"It is in that context that we must look at the history of the attack… on the theories of the cause of cerebral palsy. Sir Donald Acheson Chief Medical Officer 1983–1991, himself refers to the research into cerebral palsy, going back as far as William Little in 1862, which found that hypoxia at birth was a material cause of cerebral palsy. The hypothesis was not seriously challenged until very recently. Indeed it was the received wisdom. It is true that there were a few half-hearted attempts at research over the years but until recently all doctors – obstetricians, paediatricians and neurologists included – were prepared to accept that this was a major cause. But then the awards of damages began to increase… Suddenly there has been a flurry of research into the problem. I must say that from where I stand that seems quite scandalous. To me it is litigation/generated research and it must be suspect. …Why has there not been massive research independent of the question of accidents into a problem which is a cause of major distress to society before now? Why have there not been conferences on the causes of cerebral palsy not related to litigation? Can you see why patients and their representatives are so sceptical?"

I am bound to say that my lecture went down like a lead balloon and indeed it was one of the few occasions when I did not receive a good reception from an audience of doctors. That is hardly surprising given that I was accusing the profession of conspiracy. What is interesting is that in the main the four issues have melted away. One scarcely hears defensive medicine mentioned; cerebral palsy is dealt with on a case-by-case basis and parents are still succeeding in their claims; and risk management while of major importance in the NHS is recognised as dealing both with financial matters and patient safety. As for no-fault compensation, various schemes have been developed which deal with compensation in a different way and appear to have dampened down the demand for no fault as such. Peter Walsh, my successor as Chief Executive at AvMA discusses these in chapter 12.

However, I could not have made these points if I had not been able to see the problem of medical accidents in perspective from the victim's point of view. It was the wide experience of thousands of victims and the cases we dealt with that gave me that perspective, drove me forward and resulted in changes in the healthcare approach to patient safety, the change in attitude of the health carers and the improvement in legal procedures (and indeed the law, as I will demonstrate later). I would hear the tragic story of a patient or a relative either directly or more usually from one of our caseworkers who was appalled by what they heard and wanted me to do something about it. I would use the case, with others, to confront the health carers or contribute to a media investigation and often I could see the positive effect it had on the audience.

One of the cases I used in a lecture to midwives at the St. Mary's School of Midwifery in September 1990. The title of that lecture was Accountability and Good Practice. I often found that the best way of getting across to an audience the reality of the problems suffered by patients and the behaviour of heath care professionals was to use almost verbatim the story as related by the clients. On that occasion I used the correspondence from Mr P about his and his wife's experience on the birth of their first child. Even today, some twenty years later, it makes salutary reading so I once again quote it virtually verbatim:

"15/3/90
Further to our conversation I hereby give details of what happened to my wife after she was admitted to the Central Middlesex Hospital for delivery of our baby. She was 37 weeks pregnant at the time and it was a normal pregnancy.

28/1/90
10 a.m. Phoned the hospital because she had a 'show' and she was asked to wait until she got regular contractions.

Phoned the hospital again at 3 p.m. and told them that she was getting regular contractions every couple of hours now.

At 8.15 p.m. phoned the hospital and informed them that she was getting pains and a discharge of mucus and blood and she was told to come in to the hospital <u>if she felt like it</u>. [My underlining]

So I took her to the hospital and she was admitted at about 9.10 p.m.

At about 9.20 p.m. a foetus monitor was attached to my wife by a nurse and she was told that a midwife will come and look after her shortly.

The midwife came at 9.30 p.m. and gave my wife a physical examination and was told that my wife had dilated by 3 cms. She took the monitor off and asked my wife to walk around in the corridor so as to help with her contractions.

At about midnight she went to lay down on the bed as the contractions were getting frequent.

At about 3.45 a.m. she started getting more pains and regular contractions. So I quickly went out to the reception to look for a nurse but there was no one there.

So I went back to the room and at 4 a.m. rang the alarm. After 5 mins a nurse comes in and asks what the problem is, my wife told her that she was getting contractions every five minutes and the nurse replied that that was normal and walked out.

At about 4.45 a.m. the midwife came to the room while my wife had gone to the toilet, she said she will come back shortly.

The midwife came back at about 5.15 a.m. with a monitor and asked my wife to raise her back so that she can attach the belt for the monitor sensors. My wife said she can't move as she was in a lot of pain. At this stage the midwife examined her and noticed that the cord was hanging out.

My wife was told that they will have to do a caesarean section to deliver the baby.

My wife was rushed to the theatre and they started preparing for the operation. In the meantime another doctor comes in and suggested that they do a forceps delivery as my wife was fully dilated and the head of the baby was in the right position.

They delivered the baby at 5.35 a.m. It was a baby boy and he was not breathing on birth, he appeared completely blue in colour but his heart was still beating.

They put him on a ventilator and suction, he eventually started breathing on his own after a while and was kept on oxygen all the time.

On 3-2-90 we were told by a doctor that the baby had suffered brain damage and it was very unlikely that he will survive. I told them that I was not happy with the way my wife was neglected during labour and they suggested that I should see the consultant in charge.

On 6/2/90 I had a meeting with Mr ---- the consultant in charge and also the clinic director. I put to him the following question:

'Why wasn't my wife examined and monitored from 9.35 p.m. till 5.35 a.m.?' He said that since my wife was only in the first stage of labour so it was not necessary to monitor her. It was a busy night as well. He said that he will speak to his staff and find out what had happened and get back to me.

The baby passed away on 7/2/90 at 3.45 a.m.

On 8/2/90 I went to the Registrar's office to register the death of the baby and she asked me what had happened, she said that the coroner's office might be interested in this. So she informed the coroner's office about the situation and they said that they will take charge of the case and do an autopsy.

The coroner's officer phoned me on 9/2/90 and said that the baby had died of asphyxia which matched with what the hospital had said. He said that I can go ahead with the funeral of the baby as he had given the authorization to the funeral director. He said they are going to do a histology test which takes three to four weeks so he will contact me when the result is due. I have not heard from them since.

On 16/2/90 I had another meeting with [the consultant]. He said he was going to appoint independent advisors to investigate the hospital procedures to see if they can be improved. He said he did not have a chance to talk to the nurse who came at 4 a.m. when I rang the alarm. He said that the midwife was busy with a premature delivery that night. He agreed that if the foetus was monitored, they may have noticed that there was a problem. He said that if we decided to have another child, he will personally look after my wife and he will be present during the delivery.

I informed him that I was still not happy with his explanation and that I had left my wife in their care and they failed to look after her.

I feel that nothing will change at the hospital so I would like to take legal action against the hospital and seek compensation which may force the hospital to improve their procedures and prevent this sort of thing happening to other people."

Our case workers advised Mr P that the best way of proceeding was to arrange for him and his wife to be represented at the inquest by a barrister. There all the questions that they wanted answered would be asked and they could then decide whether they wished to proceed with legal action.

At the inquest the midwife denied that she had failed to check the mother for five and a half hours. Although the consultant had previously told the parents that the midwife was busy with a premature delivery, at the inquest he supported the midwife's version. However the Coroner did not accept their evidence. In summing up he said that he would have liked to have brought in a verdict of lack of care, but that would mean he was blaming a particular person and by law he was not allowed to do that. So he could not blame the midwife. To the consultant he said he had better go away and look at his staffing and guidelines.

That was enough for the parents. Again I think it is worth quoting from the letter our caseworkers received from them following the inquest:

"Both I and my wife have decided not to pursue this case any further as we believe that we have achieved what we set out to do... We would like to thank you for the wonderful help and advice that you have given us. We would have got nowhere at all without your assistance."

What had we done? We had, at considerable cost and distress to the parents, obtained the answers that a caring health service should have given in the first place. I am bound to say that the midwives to whom I spoke were both empathic and angry about the care that had been given and the lack of explanation.

## Growth of the casework department and how they worked

Casework was the core of AVMA. Without it, it would not have been possible for AVMA to achieve the influence it did. True, it was the lawyers whose expertise both secured compensation for victims and improved their chances of securing that compensation by forcing changes in the law and procedure. But it was AVMA's experience with the victims that enabled us to feed into the lawyers the information and training that enabled them to achieve what they did. It was also the core work of AVMA because of the large number of victims of medical accidents who needed advice and assistance. There was nowhere else for them to go.

Yet it was of course not possible to put all our resources into casework. As a result the growth of the casework department could never keep pace with demand. It was axiomatic that as the size of the department and the expertise of the caseworkers grew the backlog of cases also grew – the caseworkers were able to analyse the cases in more depth and our success brought more clients. The first person dedicated to casework, as I have recorded, was Julia Cahill. Having a medical background and also being a qualified solicitor she was able, unlike when I was dealing with the cases, to analyse the medical issues of a case as well as form a view as to whether there was a claim worth investigating.

I use the term "worth investigating" rather than "forming a view" as to whether the case had merits for a number of reasons. Firstly, given the state of knowledge of medical negligence law at that time it was quite difficult to assess a case. Secondly AVMA did not have the facilities to do the kind of work required to put ourselves into a position to decide on the merits of the case. We were not taking on legal cases ourselves so we could not apply for legal aid. While Julia Cahill could use her own knowledge of medicine to form a preliminary view it was essential that the detailed opinion of a specialist in that particular branch of medicine, based on the medical records, was obtained. We could not get that without the benefit of legal aid. So we were heavily reliant on the solicitors to whom we passed the cases to do the full preliminary work in order to decide whether a legal claim was in fact had the merits to make it worth pursuing.

From our contact with solicitors in the early days it became quite clear that the key to compensation cases was the medical issues. Given that it would be lawyers taking on the cases, Julia and I formed the view that any new caseworkers we recruited needed first and foremost to be able to understand the medical issues. If they were not legally qualified we could, with my help and the help of our referral panel lawyers, give them the necessary basic legal training so that they would have some idea of what was involved insofar as the law was concerned. I felt that the position was somewhat like the Chinese barefoot doctors. The caseworkers did not have to understand the law of property or know about criminal law or even the details of the case of Donoghue and Stevenson. (This was the case in which negligence in personal injury cases was first defined as follows: "The complainant has to show that he has been injured by the breach of duty owed to him in the circumstances by the defendant to take reasonable care to avoid such injury." It forms the basis of medical negligence claims as discussed earlier.) All they had to understand was what amounted to negligence in relation to clinical matters to be able to see whether, given a specific set of medical circumstances, there might be negligence.

Furthermore, given that it was quickly becoming apparent that what most people primarily wanted was an explanation as to what had happened to them, or their loved ones, during their medical care and that many cases would not involve the law at all, it was essential that our caseworkers should have a fairly detailed knowledge of medicine. As a result almost all the caseworkers we recruited were nurses or paramedics of some sort. Occasionally we were lucky enough to attract someone who had a legal qualification as well and from time to time we even recruited doctors. I always felt sad and a little guilty that we were taking people away from the NHS but could console myself with the conviction that firstly we would save the Health Service money if we helped to reduce accidents and secondly we were also helping people with their health. Indeed the latter was an aspect with which from time to time I berated the medical profession, stressing that a medical accident involved the health of a patient which should be of concern to them. It always seemed to me that it was as much a question of health care to ensure that someone who had suffered a medical accident received not only the additional care which might have become necessary because of the accident but also adequate financial compensation to give them as good a quality of life as was possible in the circumstances. It was because of this that I failed to understand how doctors, governed by the Hippocratic Oath, could be complicit in covering up a medical accident. I tried time and again but with limited success to persuade doctors that it was their duty not only to give explanations when asked but actually to volunteer that something had gone wrong so that immediate steps could be taken to put it right and failing that that patients could secure the compensation they needed.

I used similar arguments to try to persuade doctors to give expert evidence for victims. Whenever I could I pointed out to doctors that if they became aware that a colleague had in some way damaged a patient, whether through negligence or not, it was their duty to the profession as well as to the patient to see what they could do to help the patient. That might involve simply advising their colleague to take the necessary action to ensure that the patient suffered as little as possible, reporting the incident or giving evidence as an expert witness so that the patient could recover essential compensation.

The role of the caseworker was a heavy one. The majority of people who contacted AVMA were in an extremely distressed state. It was not simply a matter of getting the facts and advising whether legal action was a possibility. Very often the caseworker was the first person prepared to listen to the client. But if the caseworker gave the client the time that he or she needed it would mean that the number of clients that could be dealt with in a day would be very limited. I had used an answerphone from the outset when I was the only person in the organisation and clearly could not take every call. The casework department became more and more reliant on the answerphone. The message to the clients was to send in their story in a letter. Clearly that was wholly unsatisfactory from the client's point of view for a number of reasons. Firstly it was wholly unempathic. Imagine a person who has suffered a traumatic accident discovering at last that there is an organisation available specifically to help in those circumstances. They telephone and find themselves speaking, not to a kind, helpful, knowledgeable caseworker but to a machine.

Secondly it turned out to be a false economy. When the client did write in there was usually far too much information and set out in an insufficiently organised way. The record for the length of a letter to AVMA stood at 268 pages! That meant that the caseworker had to spend an inordinate amount of time trying to get to the bottom of the story. As a result the backlog of cases waiting for attention at one stage reached four months.

One of the early attempts to address these problems involved Liz Thomas. Liz came to AVMA as a temporary typist through an agency. Her background as a temp was somewhat unusual. She had a degree in pharmacology and had previously worked, among other jobs, as an Estate Agent. Secretaries at AVMA took it in turns to answer the phone when it was not in answerphone mode and though only a temp Liz took her turn with the other secretaries. She soon showed not only great intelligence but an interest in the clients about whom she was typing as well as an aptitude for talking to them on the phone. Indeed it became a problem because she was spending too much time on each call. I decided to retain her on the permanent staff – did we pay the Agency's commission? – and use her solely for speaking to clients. She had a wonderful way with them so could not only provide the support they needed but could also extract the kernel of their story. Liz's understanding of and empathy with those who had suffered, or believed they had suffered, a medical accident was an enormous asset to AVMA. She gradually rose through the ranks to become Casework Manager and then Policy & Research Manager and her influence on the development and success of AVMA cannot be overstated. At the time of writing she is still there after 20 years.

It worked to a limited extent for a while. The problem was that possibly a dozen clients received personal attention on their first call, but the number of clients was increasing relentlessly and soon the backlog grew again to an unacceptable length. Throughout my time at AVMA this problem was regularly debated by staff and Trustees. Of course the simple answer would have been to employ and train more caseworkers. But this was impossible with our limited funds. Various solutions were proposed from time to time – charge clients, limit numbers, refer straight to solicitors, close the phones from time to time.

All of these had serious downsides. I was convinced that charging clients would have changed the nature of AVMA and the relationship between AVMA and victims. We had enough clients who, having been advised by AVMA that they did not have a claim, then alleged we were simply part of the conspiracy against patients. Had we charged clients, such allegations would almost certainly have increased and would no doubt have included that we were only doing it for the money. Furthermore, I believed that victims had the right to assistance without having to pay for it. Limiting numbers would have meant that we had no control over selecting who would receive help when they most needed it and many victims would feel that once again they were being neglected. At one time or another we tried either referring clients direct to solicitors or closing the phones from time to time. Neither was satisfactory and both affected the morale of the organisation because everyone felt we were letting victims down. Although the problem was not fully resolved until after I left AVMA when it received a grant to run a Helpline we did eventually manage to reduce the backlog to acceptable limits.

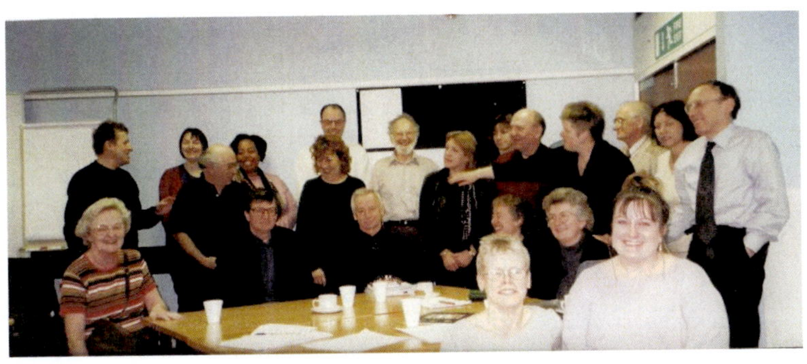

**Senior staff and Trustees 2000**

This was achieved in two ways. Firstly by the use of volunteers. From the outset, AVMA was assisted by volunteers. In the first years these were all people who had been victims and whom we were assisting. They were so grateful for having found someone who understood their problem and was trying to help them that they too wanted to help. They were happy to do anything and they were of considerable and often essential use in administrative tasks when there were only a few of us in the organisation. I even roped in my mother and my aunt, both of whom were in their seventies, to help. I am afraid that was a bit of a mixed blessing because both of them tended to distract our paid staff with constant chatter. My aunt in particular, though a highly intelligent woman, never quite got the hang of making up a file. Even in my last years at AVMA I would come across an entry in the filing book which just did not make sense. There were other volunteers who simply came in for the coffee and sympathy but even that was a bonus for our very small staff as it kept us in touch with the consequences of medical accidents. Perhaps doctors and hospital managers might have benefited from a similar experience!

Later, however, we found that trainee or newly qualified solicitors were keen to volunteer as the work at AVMA gave them first-class experience in dealing with medical negligence cases. Indeed one trainee had six months of his training contract assigned to me with the Law Society's consent. These volunteers soon learnt the ropes and although most of them worked mainly in our Lawyers' Service department, some of them were able to give invaluable support to our caseworkers.

The other way in which we almost cracked the backlog problem was by better training of the case workers so that they could identify more quickly which cases required more detailed consideration, which could not be pursued as a legal claim and which should be referred immediately to a solicitor. The training of caseworkers was a vital ingredient in the success of our casework department. Initially it was simply a case of learning on the job. Julia Cahill and I passed on our knowledge and experience to new caseworkers. Those, once they were experienced, would do the same for new caseworkers while for some time I would continue to give them formal training in the law. Unfortunately, the turnover of caseworkers over the years was quite great. The main reason for this was the nature of the work. To be faced day in and day out with the kind of tragedies they had to deal with and often to be unable to give the help that was needed led many of the caseworkers to burn out within a couple of years.

Some did stay longer and we were able to promote them to a managerial position. They could then give all the caseworkers continuous training. We were also helped by many of our panel solicitors as well as barristers with whom we worked closely. From a fairly early stage they would set up formal training sessions for our caseworkers on the law and procedure in medical negligence. As a result our caseworkers became highly expert in dealing with clients and we at AVMA always prided ourselves on our professionalism.

## The branch experiment

It was this very professionalism that led to problems when we established a branch in Manchester. In September 1984 I persuaded the Trustees that in order to reach more victims and hopefully raise more funds we should open regional branches. The idea was that we would attract a number of volunteers to form a branch management team which would then be able to raise funds locally in order to set up a fully-fledged branch. I decided to begin with Manchester because we were receiving a number of cases from that area and also because we had some excellent solicitors operating there. Roger Pannone, a partner in the firm then known as Goldberg, Blackburn & Howards (now Pannone) was a good friend of AVMA as well as being a highly competent and innovative medical negligence solicitor. (One of his innovations, however, was not so successful. In the 1980s he decided that the name of the firm was not sufficiently modern or snappy. So he took the initials and changed the name of the firm to GBH. For fairly obvious reasons the name lasted only a few months and it was changed again to Pannone & Partners.)

With the help of Roger, his partner John Kitchingman, and other solicitors we attracted a diverse number of interested people in Manchester and a Management Committee was formed. Some of the Committee members had an appropriate background, such as social work, to act as volunteer caseworkers. There is no doubt that they had the qualities to develop in the same way as the caseworkers in London had developed and had they started when AVMA was first established that would have happened. The problem was that the London caseworkers had some years' head start and had reached an advanced stage of experience and professionalism as caseworkers. Soon AVMA Manchester was attracting a stream of clients and while the Manchester volunteers were extremely diligent and caring they simply could not provide the service to clients that the professional caseworkers in London could provide.

We tried everything to maintain the branch but without funding to support a team of fully-trained caseworkers as in

London, which the Manchester Committee was unable to find, it became a drain on London. I would have to go to Manchester regularly to sort out problems and our senior caseworkers also went there frequently to try to help. But we required the volunteers to refer any slightly difficult case to London lest, through lack of knowledge of either medicine or law, they gave incorrect advice. As a result an unaffordable amount of time and money was being spent which could better have been used in improving the Head Office service. Eventually the Trustees decided that we were wasting too many resources on the branch, to the detriment of casework in London and sadly the decision was taken to close it. Notwithstanding the very clear reasons we gave those in Manchester for that step, and the fact that one of our Trustees was a retired Manchester solicitor and fully supported the decision, it did cause a certain amount of resentment and we had to work hard to ensure that that resentment did not turn into a general antipathy towards AVMA in Manchester.

Whilst that was the end of my dream of an AVMA branch in every major region it was not the end of our attempts to bring some help to the regions. Scotland was a particular problem insofar as litigation was concerned. From the outset we received a steady stream of enquiries from Scotland. Always the amount of help our caseworkers could give there was limited. Of course they could do the usual assessment as well as explain to the client what had happened and give other personal support. However, with English clients we always had the sanction of litigation. If the hospital or GP was resistant to giving information or producing the medical records we could refer the matter to expert solicitors who could issue proceedings. Often the threat of proceedings was sufficient, as the health carers in the course of time realised that the client would eventually get the information and it would simply cost them money to continue resisting.

In Scotland, however, we were up against two major problems with regard to litigation. Firstly there was a total lack of solicitors, or attorneys as they are called there, who had good experience in medical negligence litigation. We could not, of course, use our English expert solicitors because attorneys had to be qualified in Scotland to act there. Try as we might we were unable to increase the expertise of Scottish attorneys to the standard of those in

England. There were a number of reasons for this. Firstly the legal aid system in Scotland did not work in the same way as it did in England. Despite our repeated representations to the Law Society of Scotland, which dealt with Legal Aid, they would not introduce the system which we had managed to bring about in England, of issuing a Legal Aid Certificate limited to obtaining a medical expert's report. This meant that unless a client could finance a report themselves they were in a Catch 22 situation. They had to satisfy the Law Society that they had a good case in order to get a medical expert's report but until they had such a report they did not have the evidence which could satisfy the Law Society.

The second reason may also have been the result of a Catch 22 situation. In England one of the ways in which solicitors were able to increase their expertise was simply by doing more of the work as AVMA's effect on the pool of cases increased. In Scotland there did not appear to be such a large pool. That in itself may have had many causes. The Scots in general, and the medical profession in particular, put forward the hypothesis that it was because the standard of medicine in Scotland was much higher than in England so there were fewer accidents. I did buy that to some extent but later research in a large number of countries in Europe and elsewhere established that the rate of accidents in those countries was very similar so it was highly unlikely that Scotland would be unique.

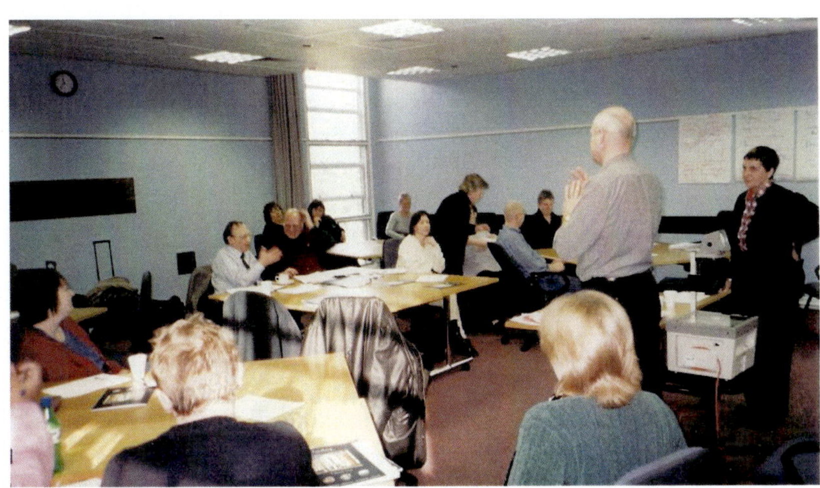

**Senior staff and Trustees training day 2000**

In any event, however, unless AVMA's influence could be felt in Scotland people who may have been victims would not come forward. And the way for AVMA's influence to be felt, as we had established in England, was to improve the success of claimants in the courts. And the way to do that was to increase the expertise of attorneys. Apart from simply doing more cases there were two ways of improving that expertise as we had learned from our experience in England. One was by training.

We ran a number of courses for attorneys in Scotland. Although a few appeared to be enthused the majority did not appear to be particularly interested. Only one or two bothered to attend our conferences in England even when they were held in the North. One of the reasons for their lack of enthusiasm appeared to me to be cultural. One of the unique aspects of the AVMA Lawyers' Service was the way in which we got solicitors to co-operate with each other. In most fields they tend to hog their expertise because of course they are in competition. Because medical negligence was a new field AVMA solicitors were only too pleased to help each other, whether it was by way of giving AVMA details of experts who had performed well or by discussing successful tactics with each other. Scottish attorneys were most reluctant to co-operate with each other, possibly because of the small number of firms as well as claimants. Thus this second way of improving expertise, learning from other solicitors, appeared to be closed in Scotland.

All this proved enormously frustrating to our caseworkers. After AVMA had been going many years they would still receive enquiries from Scottish clients whose cases had been dragging on for years or who had been told by their attorney that they had no case. On analysis it would appear that there was in fact a good case. In England the caseworker would simply have referred the case to one of our panel solicitors. In Scotland we had no panel because we were not sufficiently confident of any attorney's expertise. We did have attorneys who from time-to-time expressed a keen interest and to whom we referred all our cases. Despite dealing with a fairly substantial number of cases they did not reach the level of expertise which we felt would justify our putting them on our panel and most of them lost interest. I have no doubt that a major reason was the problems they had with legal aid.

It is interesting, however, to compare the approach of Scottish attorneys with that of solicitors in Ireland both North and South. They too had a small profession and they too had problems with Legal Aid where the system was very like that in Scotland. They had the added problem that consultants there were not prepared to act as experts. They made up for this by their enthusiasm. Perhaps because they recognised just how backward the members of the Irish medical profession were in their approach to medical accidents. Doctors there continued to have the approach that I had come up against when AVMA was first started.

But some of the worst accident cases we saw came from Ireland and perhaps that was the stimulus for the keenness of the solicitors there. Whatever the reason they, and particularly those from the South, were only too keen to learn and not only did we run courses both North and South from time-to-time but we even mounted one full-blown medical negligence conference in Dublin in February 1990, which was attended by about forty solicitors from both North and South. Following that we were able to enrol one solicitor from the North as a panel solicitor. While we had no panel solicitors in the South a number of solicitors maintained close contact with AVMA, attending conferences in England and relying on us heavily for experts.

# Chapter 10
# Casework triumphs

One of the cases which demonstrates if not dramatises almost all the aspects of AVMA's work, particularly the nature of our casework and the problems victims have had to face was that of Mrs G. Her problems started when she was diagnosed with cervical cancer. As if that were not bad enough she was treated with excess radiotherapy. The cancer was removed but awful damage was caused by the radiotherapy. She consulted AVMA in our early days when our referral panel was still in its infancy.

At that time solicitors were very dependent on barristers who had some experience in the field. The solicitors instructed such a barrister, Peter Latham. Peter was one of the first barristers if not *the* first to show a true commitment to handling medical negligence cases. So much so that AVMA invariably recommended him and he worked closely with us. I would venture to say that without Peter the cause of medical negligence litigation would have progressed far more slowly than it did. He was painstaking in his preparation of papers and extremely helpful to solicitors both in their cases and in the lectures he gave at AVMA conferences. He was prepared to, and did, push the boundaries. There were, however, two problems with Peter. Firstly, because he was so good, solicitors tended to rely on him without themselves giving sufficient thought to the merits of the case, the procedure to be adopted and the drafting of paperwork. More particularly they were prepared to wait far too long for Peter to deal with papers that he had been instructed to deal with. Which resulted from Peter's second fault. He took on too many cases as a result of which he took longer and longer in dealing with the paperwork.

Both these defects were exposed in the case of Mrs G. Peter excelled himself insofar as delay was concerned. Between the solicitors and their instructions, and the delay on Peter's part, when AVMA was finally asked to look again at the case, it turned out that five years after the writ had been served on the defendants no Statement of Claim had been served. The normal requirement for this to be done was 28 days. As a result, when the solicitors finally tried to serve the Statement of Claim the defendant's solicitors applied to strike out the claim for want of prosecution. Not surprisingly they succeeded. That meant that Mrs G could no longer proceed against the hospital involved.

By this time Mrs G's condition had deteriorated and she was not at all well. Our caseworkers gave her considerable support and having carefully looked at the facts of the case they were confident that Mrs G had a negligence case against her solicitors and barrister. This would depend on whether she could prove that it was more likely than not that her original case against the hospital would have succeeded. If that were the case, then it was clear that as a result of the negligence of her lawyers in allowing her claim against the defendants to be struck out she had lost the opportunity to receive compensation. Our caseworkers' view on her chances of success was based not only on their own assessment of the case but on the very advice of Peter Latham who had advised her solicitors, in writing, that she had a good case against the hospital which advice had ensured that Mrs G had received Legal aid to pursue that case.

At the end of the day, however, it was for Mrs G to decide whether to proceed. Unwell as she was, she was determined to see justice done. In all the developments in medical negligence litigation as well as the improvement in attitudes towards victims that have occurred since AVMA was founded, the role of victims should not be overlooked. I was always overwhelmed by the tenacity and fortitude so many of them displayed in pursuing their complaints and their legal cases. They were always aware of the enormous difficulties in doing so; the time involved; the distress in having to relate often heartbreaking stories over and over again to doctors, lawyers, tribunals and the courts; the unpleasantness of having to attack doctors and the health service which they were aware were in most cases doing fine work. To be able to do that they had to be extremely motivated. And our experience over the years was that that motivation most often did not come from the desire for compensation but from the determination to see justice done and to help to ensure that the same thing did not happen to anyone else. If it had not been for people like Mrs G, AVMA would never have been able to achieve what it has achieved.

So at the request of Mrs G the caseworker referred the case for lawyers' negligence to another AVMA panel solicitor. By this time our panel was much more rigorously monitored and we could have far more confidence in our panel solicitors. Those solicitors confirmed that Mrs G had a good case and in due course proceedings were started. Peter Latham and Ian Sheridan, the solicitor who instructed Peter, defended the case on the basis that Mrs G had not had a good case against the hospital in the first place despite the fact that Peter Latham had originally written an opinion stating that she had a good case. And this attitude was not simply an opening gambit. They pursued this defence all the way to the trial which, despite all parties proceeding with due diligence, did not take place for another three years. After a very long hearing during which the medical evidence was analysed in great detail Mrs G succeeded and was awarded compensation. Sadly, however, by this time she was a very sick woman and within two years she was dead.

The following triumph was a case which initially was referred to AVMA by a solicitor who sensibly realised that he did not have the expertise to conduct a heavy medical negligence case and asked for the name of a solicitor who did have that expertise. It demonstrates so many of the aspects of the development of medical negligence litigation that AVMA was instrumental in driving forward. In particular it demonstrates the doggedness of the defendants in resisting a claim every step of the way. We referred the case to one of our more experienced panel solicitors, Adrian Desmond of Boyes turner Burrows who reports it as follows:

> "E was born in December 1989. Things went wrong during his delivery and he was born severely asphyxiated. He went on to develop severe cerebral palsy.
>
> In August 1990 I was approached by a solicitor who was a member of E's extended family. He had been in touch with AVMA and AVMA had given him my name as a solicitor who specialised in birth injury cases.
>
> I met the family and was able to discuss issues with them initially under the then existing *"Green Form"* Legal Aid

Board Scheme. I thought that the case had merit and I therefore applied for full legal aid for E which was granted in January 1991.

1991 was still relatively early days for the direct disclosure of medical case notes and records to Plaintiff solicitors. On requesting the records the Hospital referred the matter to the Health Authorities' Solicitors, who acknowledged their interest on behalf of the Hospital at the end of February 1991 and in due course sent me the medical records.

Shortly after receiving the medical records I received a letter from Solicitors in London who acted for neighbours of E's family. They threatened the family with Court proceedings for nuisance because of what was alleged to be noise emanating from the family home caused by E's pain, distress and sleep disturbance resulting from his disability. The threats against the family were only relieved when they agreed to move to other accommodation. The obligation on my firm to assist the family as quickly as possible was very considerable but initial indications from the Hospital's solicitors were that allegations of both breach of duty and causation were to be firmly denied – and so it transpired.

I approached two Consultant Obstetricians (as was the procedure in those days). I also approached a midwifery expert, and three causation experts. All of these experts were known to AVMA and to the relatively small number of solicitors specialising in this area at that time and indeed four of those six experts continue to give evidence in these cases even today (January 2011).

The reports from the obstetric experts were received in October 1991 and March 1993. The midwifery report (commissioned a little later) was received in May 1993 and the paediatric reports in February 1992, March 1992 and June 1993.

The experts were not fully in agreement in respect of the issues of either breach or causation. Counsel who at that time was well known as a medical negligence specialist was instructed and advised on the merits of the case which enabled formal High Court proceedings to commence in

May 1992 and to be served on the Defendants' solicitors the following month. A Defence denying liability and requesting extensive further and better Particulars of the Statement of Claim were served in September 1992 and following Directions it was agreed that the matter should go forward as a split liability trial in October 1992. (That meant that there would first be a trial to decide whether the defendants were liable for the injury. If they were held to be liable then later a further trial would be held to determine how much compensation E should receive.) The claim remained firmly contested and a number of quite fiercely contested interlocutory applications (i.e. before the main trial) were heard by the Court in 1992 and 1993 before, in March 1993, the action was set down for trial at the High Court in London.

Such interlocutory applications are rare today but were very common at the time as Defendants sought to wear down the family and to test the commitment of the family's expert witnesses in particular. Also because of the urgency of the case, I commenced proceedings before all of my experts had reported to me. Whilst this was a risk, I considered it justified as it enabled me to bring the case to trial much more quickly than would otherwise have been the case.

A formal liability conference took place in May 1993 after which the Particulars of Claim were amended ahead of a liability trial scheduled to commence in May 1994.

The liability trial commenced on 9 May 1994 and ran over 9 days with the Defendants denying issues both of breach of duty and causation in which all of the expert witnesses were called.

On 28 June 1994 the Judge returned Judgment for the Plaintiff and an application for an immediate interim payment was made (and resisted). (An interim payment was necessary because E was too young for the total sum that he would need throughout his life to be quantified.)

The application for an interim payment was heard by the Court in September 1994 and an interim sum of £500,000 was awarded. A sizeable sum in those days which enabled us to purchase a property for the family. The receipt of ongoing interim payments enabled the family not only to be successfully and appropriately re-housed but also to meet E's considerable special needs.

The matter stood adjourned and E's legal aid certificate was discharged.

In October 1995 anticipating that within 2 years E's case would be capable of valuation and resolution, a new legal aid certificate was issued and quantum issues were investigated with the assistance of the experts retained on behalf of the Plaintiff.

In February 1999 the case was set down for quantum trial and was scheduled for hearing on 27 October 1999.

The Defendants' Counter Schedule (which has to set out the detailed amounts that the defendants think the plaintiff is entitled to) was received in August 1999 and the Defendants made a Part 36 payment in the sum of £2.85 million. (This is a payment of the amount the defendants say is enough to settle the claim and is a procedure designed to limit the legal costs defendants will have to pay to the plaintiffs.) The Claimant responded with a Part 36 offer of £3.5 million and the matter failed to settle.

On 27 October 1999 the quantum trial commenced and lasted for 6 days with Judgment, again reserved, being handed down on 29 November 1999 for £3.31 million some £460,000 more than the Defendant's Part 36 payment. The Defendants, continuing to resist the claim as they had consistently done over the previous decade, applied to reduce the Claimant's costs alleging exaggeration but that application was rejected."

# Chapter 11
# Working with other organisations

## Community Health Councils (CHCs)

Although CHCs were a major resource for AVMA our relationship with them was, until near my retirement, somewhat strange if not strained. CHCs were set up in 1974 to represent the interests of patients in the NHS. When AVMA was established in 1982 there was potential for conflict between the two organisations. Although it was not within their remit according to the legislation establishing them, some CHCs were quite active in dealing with patients' complaints about their health care. On the other hand, whilst AVMA's main focus was medical accidents, many complaints could be about an accident so that AVMA soon found itself dealing with complaints.

We would have been only too happy to have passed all complaints immediately to the appropriate CHC but for two problems. The first was that for many years after AVMA was established, the majority of CHCs did not deal with complaints, contending that they were not within their remit. The second was that CHC staff did not have the expertise in law or medicine to recognise when a complaint might involve a medical accident for which the patient was entitled to compensation. On the other hand some CHCs did try to give patients advice about medical negligence without having the necessary knowhow. The only solution to this was for AVMA's caseworkers to have the closest possible working relationship with those CHCs which dealt with complaints and otherwise ad themselves to help clients with their complaint.

Initially working with the first group of CHCs was difficult to achieve as most CHC staff felt we were a Johnny-come-lately treading on their toes. I personally established an excellent working relationship with The Association of Community Health Councils in England and Wales (ACHCEW), especially once Toby

Harris (now Lord Toby Harris) became secretary of that organisation. The problem was, however, that this was a co-ordinating body which, whilst providing an excellent service to those CHCs which wished to join (not all did join), could not instruct them on any matter. So they could do no more than advise CHCs that working with AVMA would be a good idea and helpful to patients.

Gradually the position improved. This was greatly helped by Toby's asking me to conduct a session on AVMA's work at a CHC Annual Conference. There I was able to explain to officers and members (at least to those who chose to attend my session which had strong competition from other sessions which many members found more relevant) exactly what AVMA was trying to do and what our particular expertise was. After that an excellent working relationship between AVMA and most CHCs developed. We regularly ran a session at CHC conferences and also set up training courses for CHCs on medical negligence. This was not intended to enable CHCs to deal with medical negligence claims but for them to be able to recognise when a complaint should be referred to AVMA. It was also agreed that AVMA would pass any complaint not involving a claim to the appropriate CHC. The symbiosis was such that when the prospect of a No Fault Compensation scheme for medical accidents was proposed in parliament by Rosie Barnes, AVMA and ACHCHEW together drafted an alternative proposal. (See chapter 8)

**The Association of Litigation and Risk Managers**

As AVMA gained status it not only improved the situation for victims but also had considerable influence on the way those acting for the hospitals and doctors approached the issue of litigation. From a situation where, before the founding of AVMA the lawyers acting for defendants could run rings around the inexperienced and often incompetent lawyers acting for plaintiffs, AVMA's panel solicitors soon became at least as good as, if not considerably better than, the defendants' lawyers. Those responsible for handling claims for hospitals and doctors and for instructing solicitors to defend claims began to realise that it was the co-operation between plaintiff solicitors that made all the difference. They realised that it would be in their interest if they too could have a means of co-operating with each other.

As a result, in 1994, Brian Capstick, one of the leading defence solicitors, founded ALARM, the Association of Litigation and Risk Managers. Jane Chapman, responsible for litigation and risk management at Northwick Park hospital became its first Chairperson. ALARM did indeed do for hospital defendants what AVMA had done for plaintiff lawyers. However there was another dimension to its work. Jane was an inspiring and sympathetic leader and very aware of the problems that victims of medical accidents suffered both in terms of their physical and mental suffering and in terms of the difficulties they had in dealing with hospitals. It was Jane's aim that litigation managers, whilst ensuring that they strongly defended defensible claims should be as open as possible with claimants and try to avoid defending claims that were indefensible.

As a result there was much common cause between AVMA and ALARM and considerable co-operation. I was invited to speak to ALARM members and Jane spoke at AVMA conferences. I recall one occasion when Jane and I shared a platform at a conference organised by one of the health organisations. I had delivered my presentation and Jane followed. She began by saying that the audience might find it surprising that she would be saying almost the same things as I had said about how medical negligence claims should be approached.

## The NHS Litigation Authority

In many ways ALARM was the precursor to the NHS Litigation Authority (NHSLA) which is a Special Health Authority set up to pool the cost of litigation and run the defences of all NHS bodies in England. Of course, being a Government body, it was much more powerful than ALARM and could not only control how cases were defended but also as part of its programme establish standards that hospitals had to abide by in order to be a member of the Litigation Authority's scheme. Like ALARM, the Authority, under its Chief Executive Steve Walker, wished to ensure that its members followed a consistent way of dealing with claims.

Steve came to see me shortly after his appointment and we had a long discussion during which I told him about the history of

AVMA, what our aims were and what we had achieved. He indicated that he was impressed and made it clear that his aims were firstly that risk management should reduce the number of medical accidents and secondly, like ALARM, he wanted NHSLA solicitors only to defend defensible claims. One of the first things that Steve did, which certainly gave me some confidence that he genuinely wanted to reduce the suffering of victims, was to issue a circular to the NHS stating that apologies did not amount to admissions of liability and therefore when an accident took place an apology should be given as soon as possible.

Unfortunately, AVMA solicitors did not always experience this new approach on the part of NHSLA solicitors. Many whose views I trusted implicitly continued to maintain that some of those solicitors were not only defending what they must have known to be hopeless cases but also behaved in an obstructive way, thus exacerbating the suffering of the victim and/or his family. This did not, however stop AVMA from developing a good working relationship with the NHSLA and I always found Steve helpful in sorting out difficult cases. In January 2008 the following extract from an article in the *Observer* demonstrated just how far Steve wanted to go in ensuring an open attitude on behalf of the NHS:

"Doctors have been told to own up and apologise if they make mistakes, in a bid to reduce the £613m in compensation paid each year to victims of blunders such as wrong diagnoses, botched surgery and delays during childbirth.

A new culture of honesty and openness should see such patients receive a personal apology from the doctor concerned and a detailed explanation of what went wrong, a senior official said. Steve Walker, chief executive of the NHS Litigation Authority (NHSLA), said that patients and their families can feel hugely frustrated when hospitals are reluctant to acknowledge and explain cases of negligence. He believes that a more candid and speedy response could reduce the £613m paid out in damages each year. He made his comments in the week that Leslie Ash was awarded £5m in damages after contracting MSSA, a variant of the MRSA superbug.

Negligence lawyers say that the main reason a number of victims take legal action is to obtain more information.

'The message to doctors is: if you're aware of an error, or a shortfall in what's been delivered, you should feel free, indeed you should feel under an obligation, to tell your patients and to apologise and to explain, either verbally or in writing, even if the patient is likely to sue,' he told *The Observer*. 'The explanation bit is really important to many, many claimants.' *It doesn't matter if it heads off a claim or encourages a claim, people as human beings and patients are entitled to this and they should be getting it.* [My italics.]

'Some patients are dissatisfied by not getting this information already. Some patients and patients' relatives feel short-changed by the system. They believe there's a lack of honesty, of frankness and of candour... I feel, and this authority feels, very strongly that people are entitled to know when something has gone wrong; entitled to an apology if something has gone wrong; entitled to an explanation of what went wrong and why, in words that they will understand; and entitled to the opportunity to ask questions about what happened and why,' Walker said. 'While some hospitals already do these things, I want to see the NHS adopt this as universal good practice.'"

On the one hand it is a sad commentary that twenty-six years after AVMA began to open up the secrecy surrounding medical accidents, medical negligence lawyers for both claimants and defendants were still saying that the main reason a number of victims take legal action is to obtain more information and this culture of openness was referred to in the *Observer* article as "new". Sad, but not surprising. In 2007 my successor at AVMA, Peter Walsh, addressed an audience of young doctors at Guys Hospital and when asked 50% said that they would not tell about an adverse incident.

On the other hand this article perfectly demonstrates how much things had changed and what a major effect AVMA has had on the issue of medical accidents and patient safety. During my time at AVMA, whenever a report came out showing the increase in the amount of compensation being paid by the NHS in respect of medical negligence – and it was always an exponential increase, never a decrease – the response by the healthcare professionals and the media was always negative. The focus was always on the damage being done to the NHS and the greed of claimants as well as the ambulance-chasing character of the lawyers. The discussion was always about how to stop people claiming and reducing the amount of compensation they could receive. Brain-damaged babies featured strongly, with the media attacking the millions of pounds paid to them without making it clear that the vast majority of that compensation went simply on helping the child to survive.

The message in this article was exactly the same as AVMA's had always been – the only way to reduce the amount of compensation is to reduce the number of accidents and when they do happen to treat victims properly.

## Defence Organisations

Whilst there are three defence organisations, the Medical Defence Union, the Medical Protection Society and the Medical and Dental Defence Union of Scotland, I mainly had dealings with the first two. The position of the defence organisations was always more difficult and more ambivalent than that of the NHSLA. The NHSLA is a government body working for the good of the NHS. As such it clearly has a duty towards the public, the users of the NHS. The role of the defence organisations is immediately apparent from their titles. It is to defend or protect doctors. Against whom one might ask? It can only be against the public.

Therefore, until AVMA came along, these organisations gave little if any attention to the needs of patients. It was always said, and indeed said to me, by trainee doctors in particular, that when representatives of these organisation came to speak to such trainees, the main thrust of their talk was to urge them as doctors to subscribe to one or other of the defence organisations (depending on which of the two the speaker came from) so as to protect themselves. To give them their due, when AVMA came along and began to berate the organisations for their attitudes they did respond. My opportunity for doing that berating usually came when I was asked to speak at conferences at which one or other of the organisations was also represented. Health conference organisers quite clearly saw the defence organisations and AVMA as representing two entirely different constituencies and that this would make for an entertaining discussion, which invariably it did – see for example my earlier reference to my talk to the Association of Surgeons in training.

I, however, saw the defence organisations as absolutely vital players in AVMA's attempts to change the attitude of doctors towards victims. After all, all doctors were urged to contact their defence organisation immediately they received a serious complaint and in excess of 90% did so. The advice the organisation then gave the doctor was crucial to how the doctor would respond to the patient. If the organisation told doctors they could, or better still urged them to, explain in full what had happened and apologise if that were appropriate the doctor would do so. But if the organisation made it clear that it was not in the doctor's interests to do so they obviously would not. This was a running battle I had with the defence organisations. The organisations, and especially the MDU, insisted that they always advised their doctors to apologise and explain. And in truth, John Wall, Secretary of the Medical Defence Union (the MDU) in the earlier years of AVMA, showed me a leaflet published by the MDU before AVMA's inception in which those very words were used. How could that be reconciled with our experience? I can only assume that when doctors actually contacted the organisation the advice was very different. Three facts remained: Firstly, that the majority of doctors believed that, as with car accidents, they should admit nothing; secondly that of the hundreds and later thousands of patients who contacted us none had received an apology or an explanation; thirdly, that John Wall's nickname as secretary of the MDU was "Wall of Silence".

So I pursued the relationship with both organisations vigorously. This was, in my view, the only way to bring about change. And to be fair, both John Wall and Roy Palmer, Secretary of the Medical Protection Society (the MPS) at that time, responded well. Interestingly it was the MDU which was initially the more co-operative. We organised joint visits to speak to medical students at which we put both sides. I do not know whether my powers of persuasion were less than before but I must admit that I was often disappointed with the attitudes of many students. Mostly they saw the MDU as their friend and

AVMA as an organisation that was pushing up the insurance fees doctors had to bear.

Later the roles of the two defence organisations were reversed. The MDU appeared to decide to plough their own furrow. The MPS on the other hand approached us to organise joint meetings and conferences and Gerard Panting from the MPS became a good friend of AVMA. He was particularly keen on co-operating with regard to mediation of claims which we both saw as promising and we worked together on that.

**The Law Society**

AVMA can truly be said to have blazed a trail with the Law Society. It seemed to me that when we started they regarded us as a unique organisation that for the first time was monitoring the quality of solicitors doing a particular type of work and, in effect, accrediting them. Whilst the Society was not at that time prepared to do anything like that themselves, I was able to persuade them that what we were doing was in the interests of both solicitors and clients. As a result they gave us a small grant to continue to run our Lawyers' Service. This was true recognition and did much to advance our status among solicitors.

Our relationship with the Law Society was always connected to the issue of Legal Aid. When we started the Law Society was in charge of Legal Aid and all our representations had to be made to them. Subsequently The Legal Aid Board (later known as the Legal Services Commission) was established to take over Legal Aid. We developed an excellent relationship with the Commission. Their legal adviser, Colin Stutt, was always willing to listen and had great respect for the work our panel solicitors did. Of course he did not always give us what we wanted but we knew that he gave serious consideration to our representations and often caused improvements to be made to the system.

With regard to our solicitor's panel and the Law Society, however, we became victims of our own success. The Society, realising the merits, and indeed the obvious sense, of having such a panel, decided to establish a medical negligence panel itself. AVMA saw this as a considerable threat to both us and victims. We had a very special way of recruiting panellists as well as a continuous monitoring system. Because we dealt with the victims themselves, we were able to see how the solicitors dealt with them and they were required to report to us regularly. With the best will in the world the Law Society would not be able to do that and we feared that their panel would simply involve a number of boxes to be ticked. There was also a concern that even the boxes to be ticked would not be sufficiently rigorous.

The threat to AVMA was also a very real one from other angles. We needed to have lawyers working closely with us in order to ensure that our clients received the very best attention and service. We were able to achieve this close relationship both because of our credibility and because clinical negligence solicitors saw it as beneficial to themselves to work with AVMA. If the Law Society panel were to become the sole arbiter of excellence and the sole route to Legal Aid it was possible that our relationship with solicitors would wither away. Given that a substantial percentage of our income came from solicitors our financial position would also suffer greatly. We saw no need for a Law Society panel and opposed its creation. We argued that they should simply give full recognition to our panel and let us continue to run it for them. For obvious reasons they could not agree and decided to go ahead. They did, however invite me to draft the criteria and procedure for membership of the panel.

That was a difficult decision for me and AVMA. However, we recognised that if there were going to be a panel, as there clearly was, we should, in the interest of victims, try to make it as effective as possible. On that basis, and on the basis that if you can't beat them, join them, my Trustees agreed that I should do it. I was able to ensure that the criteria for becoming a panel member were as rigorous as possible and that there was some monitoring of members despite the fact that those running the panel would have no direct contact with clients. I was also able to ensure that the first Director of the panel, Roger Wicks, was a solicitor with vast experience of clinical negligence who had in the past worked closely with AVMA.

One of our fears in relation to the creation of a Law Society panel was that the Legal Services Commission would recognise that panel in relation to the granting of legal aid and no longer recognise the AVMA panel. That had become extremely important as, without that recognition, solicitors would not be able to obtain legal aid for their clients. That would have been disastrous for clients. However effective I had been able to make the Law Society criteria and procedure, membership of their panel would not ensure the personal service for clients that membership of the AVMA panel could ensure. The losers would be the clients. Discussions with Colin Stutt, however, led to the decision that AVMA panel members would have equal recognition with those of the Law Society insofar as legal aid was concerned. [1]

## Mediation

One of the projects which demonstrated just how far AVMA had come in co-operating with a large number of organisations involved in litigation in one way or another was the mediation project.

Towards the end of 2000, Steve Walker, Chief Executive of the NHSLA, and I discussed the use of mediation for dealing with clinical negligence disputes. Mediation was perceived to be an excellent way to deal with some clinical negligence disputes but the number of such cases being referred to mediation was very low. AVMA could see the potential value of mediation but had certain reservations about recommending its use on a generalised and widespread basis.

Over the following months, I considered how to address our reservations and to develop procedures that would enable us to support the wider usage of mediation. Some further months of discussion and consultation between me and Steve then followed and we involved my former partner Henry Brown, a solicitor and mediator, as consultant. We concentrated on the following three areas of concern, namely:

1.  The complexities of clinical negligence disputes and the needs of the parties (both patients who had experienced clinical accidents and clinicians against whom allegations were made) which required a level of specialist expertise and skill from those mediating such disputes. If mediation were to be more widely used for clinical negligence disputes, there would need to be a significant body of specialist clinical negligence mediators with an

---

[1] The Law Society panel is now run by the Solicitors' Regulation Authority.

understanding of and sensitivity to these complexities and needs.

2. The need for a procedure that would afford parties the opportunity to explore in the particular circumstances of their case (rather than on any generalised basis) whether mediation was appropriate at that stage or at all or whether some other process, for example litigation, might be more suitable.

3. Those representing parties in the mediation process, especially the lawyers, would need to appreciate how they could best and most effectively represent their clients in the mediation process and a preliminary process review. Mediation was unfamiliar to many lawyers and this was particularly so in relation to clinical negligence cases. Not just the mediators but also the parties' lawyers needed specialist understanding and skills.

It became clear that specialist training, both of mediators and parties' representatives would be central to addressing these concerns. AVMA and the NHSLA decided that it would be essential to involve an Alternative Dispute Resolution (ADR) organisation in the development of these ideas, particularly one with a training arm and involvement in clinical negligence disputes. CEDR (Centre for Effective Dispute Resolution) was actively involved in the clinical negligence field and its Director was an experienced clinical negligence mediator. CEDR was accordingly invited to join NHSLA and AVMA in further exploring and developing these ideas.

Further discussions took place and steps were taken to seek funding for the first phase of a project to explore the practicality and viability of these ideas. It was necessary to crystallise the concepts into practical shape and to consult with a wide range of stakeholders in the field of clinical negligence disputes to establish whether there would be support for the introduction of any new procedures based on these ideas. The Legal Services Commission (LSC) agreed to fund, by way of a grant of £15,000 to AVMA and CEDR jointly, the initial phase of the project and this was approved by the NHSLA. The purpose of the funding was "to support the development of a specialist panel of senior mediators, who have advanced training and accreditation, to provide top quality mediation services in health disputes and a neutral, non-binding process consultancy to those involved in such disputes." It was also to include "a facility for lawyers and others involved in representing parties in clinical negligence cases to obtain specialised training in using mediation, evaluation, the procedural assessment consultancy and other processes effectively and constructively."

A project team was established and Henry Brown was appointed as project consultant and an Advisory Group was also established in order in order to have the views of a wide range of bodies working within the field of clinical negligence. The Advisory Group comprised the Association of Personal Injury Lawyers (APIL), the Bar sub-committee on ADR, the British Medical Association (BMA), the Clinical Disputes Forum (CDF), the Law Society of England & Wales, the Legal Services Commission, the Medical Defence Union (MDU) and the Medical Protection Society (MPS). As an important part of the consultation process, Henry Brown also contacted twelve ADR organisations apart from CEDR as well as a group of independent mediators. There was strong support for the project, for the concept that clinical negligence mediators should have specialist knowledge and skills and for a training programme for lawyers and others representing parties in clinical negligence disputes. There was also considerable support for a course that would provide specialist training for parties' representatives in clinical negligence disputes.

The project team went on to develop the idea of a process review, methods of qualification as specialist clinical negligence mediators as well as outlining the type of course that was envisaged. It was suggested that CEDR would have primary responsibility for creating the first course, which would have to be finally approved by the NHSLA and AVMA in consultation with the medical defence organisations. It was not envisaged that the proposed specialist clinical negligence accreditation would initially be an exclusive basis for the appointment of mediators in such disputes. It would though be a significant factor in the appointment, and both the NHSLA and AVMA would expect their panel members to have regard to it, while retaining freedom to appoint anyone they considered competent. Even at that time the Courts had placed an obligation on lawyers to consider the use of ADR with an increasing onus on them to do so rather than to litigate. Courts in clinical negligence cases were adjourning cases so that parties might consider ADR.

The project team was satisfied from the work done and consultation undertaken during the initial phase that the project should move forward to implementation. The problem was further funding. The LSC grant was given on the basis that the Commission would not be expected to provide further funding to the project, but would in the long term expect the project to become self-financing. Two major elements of the project were likely to be self-financing, namely the creation and presentation of the specialist mediators' training programme and the course for parties' representatives. However, it was clear that in the medium term the project would require funding to enable the various matters, apart from the creation and presentation of training courses, to be properly implemented. The initial phase of the project had crystallised the project team's original concepts into a clear and coherent programme. Unfortunately further funding was not forthcoming so the project did not proceed to implementation. However, over the years mediation came to play an important role in resolving clinical negligence claims.

# Chapter 12
# A new era for AvMA, Patient Safety & Justice:

## by Peter Walsh, chief executive of AvMA 2003–

In December 2002, having delayed his retirement in order to maintain stability at AvMA until a new chief executive could be recruited, Arnold Simanowitz finally retired after over twenty years in which he had created AvMA from scratch and developed it to be not only a lifeline for thousands of injured patients a year, but also a highly respected and influential charity. In January 2003 I became the new chief executive. This was a nervous time for AvMA and its supporters. After twenty years in Arnold's safe hands, what would happen under a new incumbent? Unlike Arnold Simanowitz, I was not a lawyer. Neither did I hold any health professional qualifications. I had been the chief officer of the Community Health Council (CHC) in Croydon (coincidentally, the town where AvMA was located). More recently, I had become the national Director of the Association of Community Health Councils in England & Wales (ACHCEW) in the middle of the highly controversial moves to abolish CHCs in England. I am told that I had gained a reputation as a tenacious advocate for both individual patients and for patients' rights in general. I believe I had also gained a reputation as a skilled and tireless campaigner during my time at ACHCEW. These were all qualities that would come in useful at AvMA, complementing the legal and medical expertise already in the organisation. However, AvMA's main support base had always been amongst the legal profession. Could I command their respect? Also, ACHCEW's campaigning against Government policy, led by me with some success, had caused considerable embarrassment for the Government. Would this baggage cost AvMA goodwill and influence in high places?

Fortunately, I inherited a strong team at AvMA who ably complemented my qualities with specialist knowledge and skills and enabled stability whilst AvMA sought to develop a new image and ways of working to make it as effective as possible in a rapidly changing environment. For all AvMA's success in getting medical accidents ("patient safety") on the agenda, which undoubtedly helped bring about radical changes such as the creation of the National Patient Safety Agency (NPSA) and a national regulator (then the Commission for Health Improvement – CHI), now the Care Quality Commission (CQC), AvMA was, due to its great success in creating a clinical negligence panel of specialist solicitors and influence over clinical negligence law, still largely perceived in many circles as predominantly a lawyers' organization, focused more on litigation than patient safety. The plan was to change that and to get AvMA recognised as a leading voice in patient safety as well as medical law, bringing a unique blend of patients' perspectives and medical and legal expertise.

One of the first challenges was to come up with a new name. The original name incorporating "victims" was felt to be a little dated. More importantly, it was perceived by doctors in particular as aggressive and failed to convey AvMA's work on patient safety. However, having built up awareness of the "AVMA" acronym, the organisation was loath to lose it. Fiona Freedland, AvMA's legal director at the time, came up with the ingenious idea of changing the name to "Action against Medical Accidents" and still using the acronym "AvMA" (with the little "v", as all lawyers would recognize, standing for "against" i.e. "versus"). With the strapline *"for patient safety and justice"* and more modern logo and livery, the change was now complete. Although the subtlety of the link between the name and the acronym 'AvMA' is lost on some, many have commented on how the change of image has helped underline AvMA's role as not only a passionate supporter of victims and the pursuit of justice, but a credible and constructive partner of all those committed to improving patient safety.

The change in image has been accompanied by a change in emphasis in the relationships with other key stakeholders. Whilst AvMA has maintained its traditional links and relationships with other key stakeholders such as claimant solicitors, the Legal Services Commission, NHS Litigation Authority and the Law Society, its relationships with the new kids on the block, the National Patient Safety Agency (NPSA) and the Department of Health itself were to become even more important. A significant breakthrough was when I was invited to join the high level

*National Patient Safety Forum.* Chaired by the chief executive of the NHS, Sir David Nicholson and the then chief medical officer, Sir Liam Donaldson, this forum brings together all the key players in the field of patient safety with the aim of steering implementation of the chief medical officer's blueprint for patient safety *"Safety First"* (*Department of Health, 2006*). The NPSA had been set up in the wake of Sir Liam Donaldson's seminal *Organisation with a Memory* and the Bristol Royal Infirmary Inquiry (to both of which Arnold Simanowitz had contributed). Its role was to collect information about things that were going wrong in healthcare, and to develop and disseminate solutions.

At about the same time a national regulator was established. Initially called the "Commission for Health Improvement" (CHI), it has already gone through various manifestations such as "Commission for Healthcare Audit and Inspection" (CHAI), the "Healthcare Commission", and subsequently the "Care Quality Commission" (CQC). Whilst AvMA had long campaigned for the establishment of an organisation with the roles played by NPSA and CQC and can justifiably claim some credit for their existence, we had envisaged the roles being within one roof. The thinking at the time the Commission was established, however, was that patient safety needed to be kept pure and completely separate from notions of regulation and accountability. Many now accept that that belief is misguided and is partly responsible for patient safety not making the advances it should have done. The problem is that whilst the NPSA did some fantastic work on understanding what was going wrong and issued good guidance to the NHS on how to reduce the risk of it happening again, it had no powers to regulate the organisations responsible for enforcing that guidance. It has to rely on a different organisation, with different governance arrangements and organisational priorities to choose to do that.

The problem was graphically illustrated by a high profile report published by AvMA in 2010 – *Adding Insult to Injury: NHS Failure to implement Patient Safety Alerts*. AvMA sought information under the Freedom of Information Act on the number of NHS bodies who had declared compliance with all 53 patient safety alerts which had been issued since the NPSA's inception, for which the deadline for completion had already passed. Patient Safety Alerts are only issued about the most serious issues after careful consideration of all the evidence and consultation with experts. They are usually matters quite literally of life and death, and timely implementation of them is one of the top 'core priorities' laid down by the Department of Health for the NHS. The results were shocking. Hundreds of trusts had not implemented at least one alert and 80 had not implemented 10 or more alerts, some going back as far as five years. One trust had failed to implement 37 out of the 57 alerts! However, even more shocking was the fact that no one body took responsibility for monitoring and chasing up trusts who had not complied. The NPSA said that this was beyond their remit. They had done their job by developing and disseminating the alerts. The CQC which does, as a regulator, have the power to play this role, had other priorities such as concentrating on its registration process and a sophisticated system for analysing a raft of "risk factors" in the performance of healthcare organisations. When AvMA pressed them on a response as to how they were dealing with the simple fact that information was currently available to them, showing that NHS trusts were putting patients' lives at unnecessary risk by failing to implement the alerts, they admitted that they were doing nothing.

However, this is a perfect example of how AvMA can provide a reality check on how, what on the face of it seems a very credible system, works in practice, and can help bring about improvements. Helped by widespread media coverage, AvMA succeeded in getting the Department of Health to issue a letter to all trusts reminding them of the need to comply with alerts and the CQC at least to write to trusts that are not compliant, to ask them to explain and say when they will be. The dangers of the system not being "joined up" are all too plain to see, and it could well be that moves will be made to join up the system. At the time of writing, the coalition government faces the toughest economic environment for decades. We can only hope that we may yet see the roles of promoting patient safety and the regulation remain a top priority. As discussed later, the signs are not good.

A common thread through the whole of this book is AvMA's quest for a genuinely open and fair culture, where health providers are always open with patients and their families when things go wrong that have caused harm or may result in harm developing in the future; where the system learns from such incidents so as to make treatment safer for other patients; where health professionals are not inappropriately blamed for genuine individual mistakes or system failures or for being honest with patients or "whistleblowing"; and where patients or their families are compensated fairly for their avoidable loss due to sub-standard treatment. The term "open and fair culture" has now become the common vocabulary in the patient safety world, at least in the United Kingdom. Initially, at about the time the NPSA was being set up, the phrase most commonly heard was "no-blame culture". This became a mantra for health professionals who felt persecuted for all of healthcare's failings and the so-called "compensation culture" and for many others in the patient safety movement. Many would say that the phrase was hi-jacked. Certainly, it has been misunderstood or misused to suggest that health professionals should be protected from normal accountability, or even that it might be legitimate to withhold information about a medical accident from patients or their families.

At a high profile conference hosted by the British Medical Journal as late as 2005, one well known patient safety expert from Australia proudly told the audience (almost completely made up of health professionals and managers) of the patient safety incident reporting system used in his state. He gave the example of how the system received a report from an anaesthetist about an incident where the patient died during surgery as a result of the anaesthetic equipment not operating properly. It had not been checked before surgery. As a result of looking further into the issue, lessons were learnt and guidance issued about the fault that had occurred and about pre-operative checks. When I, who happened to be in the audience as one of the forthcoming speakers, asked whether the patient's family had been informed, the learned doctor replied, without a hint of embarrassment, "no". His view was that if his colleague thought that the family would come to know that this death was perfectly avoidable and that he or she might be held to account for what had happened in any way – to suffer from the "blame culture" – he would never have provided the report, even to the reporting system. Although he acknowledged that it seemed unfair that the family should never know, it was for the greater public good that the system received the information. What was so striking about this was that although in the break I was warmly congratulated by several attendees for challenging the ethics of this approach, the vast majority of the audience simply accepted it as common sense or even the norm.

In other debates, the airline industry is still quoted *ad nauseam* for its successful approach to safety and in particular its reporting system, which protects the reporter of incidents from blame. What the proponents of this approach often fail to recognise or acknowledge are two simple facts. Firstly, an obvious difference between a pilot and a doctor is that a pilot goes down with his or her plane. Secondly, while the airline industry protects reporters of "near miss" incidents from blame, it would be completely unthinkable in the airline industry for an incident which had caused actual harm to a passenger, to be swept under the carpet. Yet for some, healthcare is different in that respect. More than any other organisation, it continues to be AvMA that challenges the *status quo* and keeps the ethics of how to manage the aftermath of a medical accident on the agenda. There has been some success so far, at least on the face of it, when it comes to "being open". At least the rhetoric has changed. For "no-blame culture" read "fair blame" or "open and fair" culture. Thanks to lobbying by AvMA, the NHS Constitution now contains a principle of being open and honest with patients when things go wrong (something that was not there in the draft that went out for consultation).

AvMA also scored a notable success (albeit at the temporary cost of relationships with the NHS Litigation Authority ) with getting the guidance issued by that authority changed in 2009. Since 1997, the NHSLA had boasted of what it considered to be an enlightened approach to offering explanations and apologies to patients when things went wrong. It issued a circular (referred to earlier) on the subject to all NHS trusts which, to be fair, was probably quite radical and enlightened at the time it was first issued. In fact, my predecessor Arnold Simanowitz commended it because for the first time health professionals were told that offering an apology did not necessarily amount to an admission of liability. It talked about trusts offering "apologies" and "explanations" – something which some insurers still shy away from, preferring the "admit nothing, say nothing" approach. In 2009 the circular was due to be freshened up and re-issued. AvMA expressed grave reservations about the wording which almost entirely drew on the original. Whilst on the face of it encouraging apologies and explanations, a closer reading revealed some fundamentally outdated thinking and even, potentially, a cynical approach. An apology was defined merely as an "expression of regret at an outcome" or "sympathy" about what had happened. In AvMA's experience, it is precisely this sort of approach that does more harm than good. Nothing was mentioned about accepting responsibility – something people commonly understand as constituting a *meaningful* apology. Someone expressing sympathy or regret that one of your loved ones had died or been grievously harmed without acknowledging that their organisation may have avoided this, if that is the case, is like a red rag to a bull to those injured or their relatives and immensely hurtful.

Even worse, the circular went on to issue a stark warning to trusts that in doing all of the above "care must be taken to avoid future litigation risks". In other words, be sympathetic by all means and offer explanations up to a point, but don't give the patient information which might help them if they take legal action to obtain compensation. Hardly enlightened thinking by today's standards! In spite of the concerns AvMA expressed and its offers to help draft a more suitable version, the NHSLA were to re-issue the circular practically unchanged except for the endorsements of various health professional and defence bodies, until AvMA intervened at the National Patient Safety Forum and the chief executive of the NHS told the NHSLA it could not go out as it was. Eventually, a revised version with AvMA's suggestions included was issued, which was some achievement. It now said all the right things. However, the fact that it had been such a struggle and the NHSLA were forced into changes does raise questions about how much insight and ownership of the new approach really exists.

The NPSA showed much more willingness to engage when it developed its *Being Open* guidance in 2006. AvMA and other stakeholders were fully consulted and the result showed that they had been listened to. One of the significant changes was the change in title from "Open Disclosure". Although this is the term most widely used internationally for informing patients or their relatives about things that go wrong, it was felt that the term both sounded too legalistic and implied that health providers were the owners of the information and that it was an issue as to whether it should be "openly disclosed". The alternative is that any information about what happens in a patient's care is legitimately theirs. Now, as "Being Open", the guidance is widely accepted as being excellent and was even refreshed and re-issued in 2010. However, it remains only guidance. It is hardly surprising then, given the pressures faced by NHS trusts to achieve numerous compulsory targets, implementation of the guidance has been found to have been given relatively low priority and is patchy to say the least. The health professional bodies and defence organizations have thus far been successful in lobbying against any compulsion to do the right thing when it came to dealing with patients who had been harmed. Whilst everyone seems to agree that "being open" is the right thing to do, at least in theory, to some it is not as important as the many "must do's". To them, it is a question of appealing to hearts and minds and waiting for a change of culture – however long that takes. In the meantime, they are prepared to accept that the culture of denial and cover-up goes on. AvMA however, continues to make the case that so fundamental an issue needs to be underpinned by law.

AvMA had long called for a legal or statutory duty to be open with patients. An increasing number of countries around the world have taken this step. In 2003 the Chief Medical Officer Sir Liam Donaldson formally recommended a legal "duty of candour" in his report *Making Amends* (Department of Health, 2003). To this day, there has never been a credible explanation of why this step has not been taken. The best ministers at the time could come up with was that a professional duty to be honest already exists within the professional codes of bodies such as the General Medical Council (GMC). However, it can be safely assumed that the chief medical officer and his officials fully understood that such a professional duty existed when they drafted the recommendation and believed it was not enough. The codes themselves are discretionary, and only apply to health professionals registered with that body. There is no equivalent duty against which other health managers and staff or organisations corporately can be held to account. Even where well-evidenced allegations of dishonesty and cover-up were available to the GMC, they could not be relied upon to take action. In 2008 AvMA decided to take the unprecedented step of taking legal action itself to challenge a decision of the GMC not even to investigate allegations against several GPs accused of attempting to cover up mistakes leading to the avoidable death of ten-year-old Robbie Powell in South Wales, by falsifying medical records. His father, Will Powell had struggled bravely for years to hold these doctors to account. In spite of the length of time that had elapsed through no fault of his own, the evidence remained fresh and available and if the allegation were true, these doctors were both continuing to practise and to continue the cover-up. The Local Health Board in which they worked itself, as well as AvMA and others asked the GMC to investigate. Yet, the GMC decided not to, by invoking its "five-year rule" and refusing to use its discretion to waive it. It argued that even if the allegations were true, it was not sufficiently in the public interest or an exceptional enough set of circumstances to waive the rule which protected the doctors from even being investigated. AvMA won permission in the High Court to take the issue to judicial review in spite of fierce resistance from the GMC. However, the case was withdrawn when the GMC succeeded in having AvMA's protected costs order taken away, thus effectively threatening the charity with bankruptcy if it went to court and lost. The message of the GMC's stance appeared to be that even well-evidenced allegations of cover-up were not important enough to waive their five-year rule for. The longer doctors are successful in covering up therefore, the less likely they are to be investigated.

The experience of this judicial review both increased AvMA's determination to obtain a legal duty of candour and served as an inspiration for developing its approach to casework in the future. AvMA's campaign for the legal duty of candour became known as the campaign for "Robbie's law" in honour of the family's heroic struggle, and gained pace. By the time of the general election in 2010, the Liberal Democrats had included it in their manifesto, albeit in a form of words that would prove to be crucially flawed. The commitment was to "require hospitals" to be open when things go wrong. Presumably this was drafted by a public relations person who felt the man and woman in the street needed things kept simple. As a result of the formation of the coalition government, the commitment became part of the coalition's "programme for government" and was included in their White Paper *Liberating the NHS*. However it quickly became apparent that the Conservative half of the coalition did not appreciate what in principle they had committed themselves to. There was silence about how this new "requirement" would be put in place. Nothing appeared in the draft Health and Social Care bill about it. When AvMA pressed the issue with the ministers responsible for this area (who were Conservative) the ideological chasm became clear. They were ideologically opposed to introducing any new statutory regulation, and particularly over this. The impression I had was that they would not do anything at all on this issue if they could get away with it, but faced with an increasingly powerful campaign headed by AvMA and supported by leading national patients' groups and many others including health professionals, managers and patient safety experts, they simply had to do something. The Health bill had a tortuous passage through parliament for a host of reasons and at one point came to a halt to conduct a listening exercise with all key stakeholders. There was widespread support, particularly, but not exclusively, from patients' groups to introduce a statutory provision for a duty of candour in the Bill itself. AvMA was working with parliamentarians on an amendment to do just that, which was clearly going to attract a lot of support in the House of Lords at least.

Faced with all of this, the Department of Health announced its own proposals for a "Duty of Candour" which went out to consultation. However, this "Duty of Candour" was only to apply to NHS Trusts (mainly hospitals), explicitly omitting general practice, and was to have no statutory force. It was proposed that it would take the form of a standard clause in trusts' contracts with the new Clinical Commissioning Groups. Had the original wording of the Liberal Democrat manifesto commitment which became part of the coalition agreement been better worded (by not using "hospitals" as a generic term for the NHS, and by specifying that the "requirement" would be statutory) perhaps they could not have got away with such a proposition, which seemingly failed to please anyone. In any case an amendment to introduce a statutory Duty of Candour in the Health Bill was debated in the Lords. Most commentators agreed that the debate was "won" in favour of a statutory duty, but because of a three-line whip applied by the Government the vote was lost. Bizarrely, Liberal Democrat peers, even those who had supported and put their names to the amendment, voted against it. Had only a few even abstained it would have been carried and (if the Commons did not overturn it) would have represented the biggest advance in patients' rights and patient safety since the formation of the NHS. As it stands at the time of writing, it will remain the case that there is no statutory obligation on healthcare organisations to tell a patient or their family about incidents which have caused harm to the patient under their care. This issue will be returned to at the end of this chapter when we look to the future.

The judicial review of the GMC also fuelled AvMA's desire to align its casework more with its campaigning priorities. Having established the specialist clinical negligence panel of solicitors and an ongoing programme of training and developing specialists in medical law, AvMA's focus with its own casework shifted more to where it could add special value. In 2008, ten families who had lost loved ones at Gosport War Memorial Hospital heard there would finally be an inquest into their deaths in the late 1990s, which were among hundreds due to extraordinary use of diamorphine and which were shrouded in controversy. None of the families could find legal representation at the inquest and so AvMA offered to bring families together to discuss shared objectives and tactics. Using its relationship with specialist lawyers in its membership, AvMA secured the services of Blake Lapthorn – a local firm – who offered to represent the families without any funding being available. (In the event, some legal aid was secured, but not until the inquest had started.) The inquest findings vindicated the long campaign by families to get to the truth behind the deaths. Subsequently, the GMC finally took action against the GP at the centre of the scandal. The case underlined the problem with lack of representation for families at inquests into healthcare-related deaths. AvMA finds that this is not a problem where there is a likely clinical negligence claim to follow. Solicitors will generally take these cases on. However, if it is a case where it is not obvious there is a claim it can be very difficult to get legal representation, whereas the trust, doctors and nurses will always have heavyweight representation. This can make it very difficult for families to have any meaningful involvement in what is a vitally important opportunity not only for them but also for the system to learn more about the reasons for the death and whether similar deaths can be avoided.

As a result of AvMA's growing concern about the problems with inquests and its desire to focus its energy and expertise more strategically where they can add most value, AvMA set about developing a service specifically to support families with healthcare related inquests. Although no funding was available to develop this service, AvMA directed much of the modest resources it had to plugging this gap and due to the tremendous goodwill of solicitors and barristers in AvMA's network, were able to get them to offer *pro bono* representation where it is needed.

Some of the first cases taken on underlined the importance of inquests. One of the worst, if not the very worst ever hospital scandal came to the surface in March 2009 as a result of the Healthcare Commission (now the 'CQC') report into Mid Staffordshire NHS Foundation Trust. It estimated that potentially hundreds of patients died prematurely due to the appalling standards of care at the trust. AvMA reacted quickly both to offer its support to families affected by the scandal and to call for a public inquiry into how, with all the structures that were in place, this could have been allowed to happen. Several families needed representation at inquests and more needed support and advice in going through the independent case note reviews that the then Secretary of State, Alan Johnson, offered them. AvMA was the only agency able to provide this kind of specialist support, and devoted large amounts of staff time to the project. However, the Government steadfastly refused to call a public inquiry, instead opting for a limited inquiry tightly restricted by the terms of reference it set. Notably, the inquiry was to be restricted to events at the hospital and not look at the wider picture such as the Department of Health itself, and the systems it had put in place which were meant to prevent this kind of thing happening. AvMA continued to work with the hugely impressive local campaign group, Cure the NHS in Stafford, to demand a full public inquiry, and both opposition parties at the time promised one, should they come to power. Sure enough, when the coalition government was formed, a full public inquiry with the terms of reference AvMA and Cure had been calling for was opened. AvMA was to play a central role in it, representing the interests of the wider public and placing its knowledge of national systems of patient safety, regulation, complaints, and public engagement at the disposal of the inquiry. At the time of writing, the report of the inquiry which was chaired by Robert Francis QC was eagerly awaited and may have big implications for the future.

Although the charity has successfully repositioned itself to be seen and accepted as a credible patient voice on patient safety, it has in no way diluted its commitment to access to justice. AvMA has been rightly accorded much of the credit for improvements in the way that clinical negligence litigation and medical law works over the years and improving access to justice for people harmed by medical accidents. In the 1990s it had succeeded in fending off proposals to scrap legal aid for clinical negligence cases and ill thought out proposals for so-called "no-fault compensation" schemes. Whenever these came to be looked at in detail the terminology seemed misplaced. Almost invariably there is a requirement to demonstrate "fault". Indeed, it would be illogical to compensate someone when there had not been any fault.

Such schemes also tend to under-compensate people – leaving them without the level of compensation they genuinely need and deserve – in order to "lower the bar" and offer more limited compensation to a greater number of people. The Chief Medical Officer, Sir Liam Donaldson, considered alternatives to litigation in his review leading to the publication of *Making Amends (2003)*. Whilst this did contain a recommendation for a no-fault compensation scheme for brain-damaged babies, this was eventually ditched as being impractical. The recommendation for an NHS Redress Scheme (an administrative scheme to offer financial and other redress in lower value "claims") was taken forward by the then Labour Government who eventually passed the NHS Redress Act (2006) to create a scheme, only to allow it to gather dust on the shelf. The proposals were not perfect but during the passage of the legislation AvMA managed to secure various concessions which meant that it would have offered a viable alternative to litigation for many people with what would be lower value claims of up to £20,000. Some of these are extremely serious, often fatal cases which are not amenable to litigation because of the limited damages on offer.

AvMA has always argued that there are better ways than litigation to give people the compensation they need and deserve and also ensure lessons are learnt, as was demonstrated with the "Resolve" pilot scheme run with the NHS Litigation Authority and an insurance company called Litigation Protection. This pilot small-claims scheme in which AvMA played a pivotal part, sought to resolve these claims without the need for litigation. Thanks to

AvMA, it also attempted to "close the loop" between the incidents resulting in claims and learning for patient safety. However, to this day such approaches remain just an aspiration. It should be noted however that a second look at the possibility of a "no-fault compensation" scheme for medical negligence in Scotland commissioned by the Scottish Government and in which AvMA took part did recommend a "no-fault" scheme in Scotland. Frankly, access to justice through medical negligence litigation is so limited in Scotland that almost anything would be an improvement. However, the Scottish Government has still not committed itself to introducing such a scheme even though it is official policy to do so. Ironically, the Welsh Assembly Government did decide to enact powers it was given by the NHS Redress Act 2006 to set up its own redress scheme. Contained within the wider provisions of its "Putting Things Right" initiative, it was launched in April 2011. It seems to have had mixed reviews but it is too early to tell if it can prove itself to be a satisfactory alternative to litigation.

During the first decade of the century the costs of clinical negligence litigation continued to grow. Legal Aid gradually declined as the main funding source for clinical negligence claims with conditional fee agreements (CFAs) taking over that position. This was a direct consequence of government policy, which constricted eligibility for legal aid more and more. Many solicitors also preferred the freedom that CFAs provided. In addition, CFAs allowed for generous "success fees" in successful cases. Solicitors became more and more adept at running and winning cases on CFAs. One consequence of that was an exponential increase in legal costs associated with clinical negligence due to the high success fees and cost of medical expert reports. Whilst talk of a so-called "compensation culture" when it comes to clinical cases was very ill-informed or mischievous (it is well established that people are reluctant to sue in these cases and far fewer do than have reasonable cause to), there is no denying something had to change.

A Labour government had already instructed the Right Honourable Lord Justice (Rupert) Jackson to review civil litigation. His report *"Review of Civil Litigation Costs"* (The Stationery Office, 2009) was radical enough, recommending huge changes to the way CFAs worked. However, no one really expected quite how dramatic the changes that were to come would be. AvMA was to face a gigantic challenge in seeking to limit the damage to be caused by the overhaul of the civil litigation system contained in the Legal Aid Sentencing and Punishment of Offenders Act (2012). Faced with the economic crisis and the need to make cuts, but also an ideological zeal fuelled by myths about "compensation culture" and an innate dislike of legal aid in some parts of the Government, it was proposed not only to change the way that conditional fee agreements work, but to scrap legal aid for clinical negligence cases. This incidentally was something which Lord Justice Jackson himself was strongly and outspokenly against. He was clear that his proposals for reforming CFAs were based on legal aid being retained. This is not the place for an analysis of the pros and cons of the new arrangements, but suffice to say that in AvMA's opinion they are both deeply damaging to access to justice and irrational, in that they are unlikely to lead to any real savings for the tax payer. Something that was lost on many of the politicians was the fact that use of legal aid, according to all the evidence, had been by far the most cost effective way of settling clinical negligence claims. Many millions of pounds had been wasted by the insistence by successive governments on preferring conditional fee agreements (no-win no-fee) as a method of funding. The exponential increase in costs because of insurance premiums and success fees was inevitable, and a direct result of government policy. Something did need to be done to curb the excessive costs associated with litigation, but with clinical negligence in particular the most logical solution would have been to allow legal aid for all cases. However, that would have been politically incorrect.

Whilst the Act impinges on many areas of law and faced stern resistance from all quarters, AvMA's was the only voice specifically concentrating on clinical negligence. Enormous effort was put into trying to bring about changes to protect access to justice for some of the most needy and deserving cases in society. Once again however, it had won all the moral and logical arguments without achieving the desired changes. The charity was widely quoted and its briefings praised in the debates over this part of the Bill but such was the Government's determination to press ahead whatever the evidence and counter arguments, key votes were lost. A key vote on an amendment in the House of

Lords which would have preserved legal aid for clinical negligence was lost by just seven votes late at night following filibustering by Government peers. Once again, Liberal Democrat peers expressed their sympathy and support in principle but followed a three-line whip.

## The Future

2012, the 30th anniversary year of AvMA, represented another watershed in its history. The effects of the Health and Social Care Act and the Legal Aid Sentencing and Punishment of Offenders Act will have profound implications for patient safety and access to justice for years to come. One consequence of the Health Act is the disappearance of the National Patient Safety Agency (NPSA). While the NPSA was not perfect, it was internationally respected and the loss of its pure focus on patient safety may come to be regretted. The context of this change was the need to save money. The resources previously applied to its work will not be available to the NHS Commissioning Board, into which it is planned it will be subsumed. The NHS as a whole is having to cope with huge challenges with no increase in resources. The financial squeeze may result in a watering down of the resources deployed towards patient safety – however short-sighted that would clearly be. Coupled with that, reorganisation in the NHS inherently increases risk and the wider changes brought about by the Act are huge. Once more patient safety appears to have taken a back seat. There appears to be an assumption that the "C" words – competition and commissioning (which some see as a pseudonym for privatisation) will somehow make things better, but without any evidence to support the theory. Patient safety does not appear to have featured in the risk assessment of the reforms at all according to the leaked version of the Government's risk assessment obtained by *The Guardian*. (The Government refused to publish the risk assessment even though the Information Commissioner had ruled that they should!) A key challenge for AvMA will be to keep patient safety high on the agenda and to continue to probe and challenge when this is not the case. Similarly, access to justice for the people AvMA serves is severely under threat, potentially putting back years of achievements in this area. Some people have questioned whether as a result of the loss of legal aid for the vast majority of cases, there is a future for the AvMA panel of specialist solicitors. (Panel status is used by the Legal Services Commission as a requirement for a franchise for legal aid in clinical negligence cases.) However, AvMA is firmly of the view that the panel will be needed even more under the new system. The public will be confronted by a bewildering range of solicitors and claims farmers offering 'no-win no-fee' arrangements, but without the required expertise (just like the old days). A major campaign is planned to make the public aware of AvMA's quality mark for specialist solicitors and help them avoid the risks of dealing with non-specialists.

Although AvMA's support for "victims" of medical accidents has developed hugely since the early days, AvMA will have to seriously rethink how it provides its own services so as to ensure gaps in advice and representation provision are met, and AvMA concentrates on where it can best add value. AvMA's helpline (which currently serves over 3,000 people a year) will always be a vital point of contact for people affected by a medical accident, providing a knowledgeable and sympathetic response, explaining options and rights, and helping people make informed decisions about what to do next. Thanks to the specialist clinical negligence panel, where a clinical negligence claim is a desired option, people can be fast-tracked to a suitable solicitor. However, where AvMA may be better placed to provide or arrange suitable support or representation, AvMA itself can be more involved. For example in inquests concerning healthcare related deaths which is an area in which AvMA has had great success recently in targeting its casework; in referring cases to the fitness to practice procedures of the GMC or NMC (Nursing and Midwives Council); in system failures involving large numbers like Stafford; or where the case links to a campaigning priority for the charity such as cases involving cover-ups. Like a lot of charities, AvMA has always been able to help more people by bringing about changes in systems than it could ever do through the direct support it provides to individual cases. It now has a model that aligns its direct support to members of the public with its strategic priorities for bringing about improvements to patient safety and justice. AvMA will continue to work in partnership with others and where necessary campaign, as well as provide direct services.

The recommendations from the Mid Staffordshire NHS Foundation Trust Public Inquiry, when they are published, may provide new opportunities for AvMA to push for much needed improvements in patient safety. Given the weight of evidence heard by the inquiry on the need for a statutory duty of candour and the apparent interest in that of the chairman and counsel to the inquiry, it is likely that the report will have something to say about it. Achieving the real, meaningful, statutory Duty of Candour will remain a top priority for AvMA as it goes to the very heart of what the charity is about. The position whereby cover-ups are frowned upon but tolerated is unsustainable. Whilst no rule or law on its own changes culture or behaviour, without it the long-aspired change of culture simply won't happen – justice will continue to be denied and lessons will not be learnt for patient safety.

Patient safety and justice and AvMA face an uncertain future, but one thing is certain: the need for AvMA, in spite of its many achievements, firmly remains. One of the greatest uncertainties for AvMA has always been its funding. The charity receives no core funding from other agencies and over the years has had to survive on the occasional one-off grant, its own efforts to raise funds by putting on top quality conferences and providing advice and information services to lawyers, and the generosity of its supporters. Each year has been under the shadow of whether there will be the resources available to continue the work for another year (leading to considerable loss and greying of hair for both the first and the current chief executive!)

However, something wonderful happened to AvMA in 2011 which means that it can plan for the future in a way it has never had the opportunity to do before. A previous client who had contacted AvMA for advice years ago chose to remember AvMA in her will. Ironically, the volume of work that AvMA did on her case was very small in comparison to the average, but she was so impressed with the fact that such a body actually existed she chose to make AvMA the main beneficiary, and such was the size of her estate that the charity is planning to purchase its own office accommodation as a means of securing the ongoing viability of the charity and planning to expand rather than cut back, as would have been the case without the legacy. That woman was Judith Freedman – a renowned social anthropologist. It is only fitting that her name should be remembered alongside those other giants of patient safety and justice like the founding fathers of AvMA, Arnold Simanowitz OBE and Peter Ransley.